The Ergonomic PC
Creating a healthy computing environment

Baird Peterson
Richard Patten, CHFP

McGraw-Hill

New York   San Francisco   Washington, D.C.   Auckland   Bogotá
Caracas   Lisbon   London   Madrid   Mexico City   Milan
Montreal   New Delhi   San Juan   Singapore
Sydney   Tokyo   Toronto

©1995 by **Baird Peterson and Richard Patten**.
Published by McGraw-Hill, Inc.

pbk   1 2 3 4 5 6 7 8 9 0 FGR/FGR 9 9 8 7 6 5

Library of Congress Cataloging-in-Publication Data
Peterson, Baird.
    The ergonomic PC : creating a healthy computing environment / by
Baird Peterson, Richard Patten.
        p.   cm.
    Includes index.
    ISBN 0-07-049664-1   (pbk.)
    1. Microcomputer workstations—Health aspects.   2. Human
engineering.   I. Patten, Richard.   II. Title.
RC965.V53P48   1995
651.8'401'9—dc20   95-16760
                                                             CIP

Editorial team: Jennifer Holt DiGiovanna, Acquisitions Editor
              Michael Christopher, Book Editor
              David M. McCandless, Managing Editor
              Joanne Slike, Executive Editor
Production team: Katherine G. Brown, Director
              Brian Allison, Computer Artist
              Wanda S. Ditch, Desktop Operator
              Joann Woy, Indexer
Design team: Jaclyn J. Boone, Designer   WK2
              Katherine Stefanski, Associate Designer   0496641

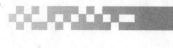
The Ergonomic PC

998

9

000

To Maureen and Colin.   *B.P.*

To Dorothy, Jim, Sonia, Steve, Chris, Alex, and Rocky.   *R.P.*

Contents

Part 2
Working conditions

Acknowledgments

I give my heartfelt thanks to my wife, Maureen, and son, Colin, for their patience during my hours and hours of writing. I also thank Paul Turgeon, Barbara McMillan, Peggy Bauer, and Geanne Whetstone for gathering many articles and books for this project.   *Baird Peterson*

I thank Sonia, Alex, Chris, and Rocky for their patience during my writing. I also thank Cathy O'Brien, OTR, CHT, for reading my material about cumulative trauma disorders. I thank Brad Zadnam—Senior Research Analyst with the Minnesota Department of Labor—who gave me important information about the history of worker's compensation law. Colleagues Ray Wahlgren and Jim Kochevar deserve thanks —Ray for wise counsel and Jim for providing photographs.   *Richard Patten*

We both thank our editors at TAB/McGraw-Hill for their skill and patience. We also thank our anonymous reviewers for their valuable advice.

The Minneapolis Public Library, the Hennepin County Library, and the University of Minnesota library gathered hundreds of books and articles that we used when we wrote *The Ergonomic PC*—and we thank all three library systems.

We thank the U.S. Chamber of Commerce for permitting us to reprint some of their material in an appendix. We also thank the journal *Spine* for permitting us to use figures from articles by Andersson *et al*.

Introduction

The Ergonomic PC is for anyone who uses a computer or manages other workers who do. Either way, the book will help you keep yourself—and anyone else who works for you—healthier and more productive.

Chapters 1 through 4 tell you about the medical problems that a poorly designed chair can cause. You'll learn how to choose and use a chair that will boost your productivity and help to protect you from injuries. You'll also learn the importance of diet, regular rest periods, movement, and exercise in defending yourself against the health problems that prolonged sitting can cause.

Chapter 5 tells you what features you should look for in a workstation. It tells you how poorly designed workstations can cause vision problems and upper-body pain. It also tells you how to recognize the poor keyboarding technique that makes cumulative trauma disorders such as carpal tunnel syndrome more likely. It shows you ways to make it safer for you to use a keyboard.

The chapter also mentions the obligations of employers in connection with workstations, under the recent Americans with Disabilities Act (ADA).

Chapter 6 discusses computer workstation standards in relation to potential OSHA regulations. Chapter 7 gives you tips for reducing worker's compensation costs. Chapter 8 reviews the controversy about radiation from video displays.

Chapters 9, 10, and 11 tell you some easy ways to boost your productivity and make your work more enjoyable—and do the same for anyone who works for you. You'll also learn how to justify your need—and your workers' needs—for quiet and privacy. The chapters also tell you how to choose video displays to minimize glare and eyestrain and how to arrange lighting to further reduce glare.

Chapter 11 tells you how to boost your organization's productivity with groupware. It also tells you what changes in your organization you should expect after you start using groupware. A manager's checklist tells you how to get the biggest benefits from your groupware investment with the least trouble.

Chapter 12 explains the importance of using high-speed hardware and software for your computer work. It gives you valuable information that you can use to justify your investments in high-speed hardware and software. It also gives you practical tips for increasing the speed of your hardware and software.

Chapter 13 tells you the single, most important step that most users can take to boost their productivity when they use a computer. It tells you what features you can reasonably expect to find in a high-speed word processor—so that you won't make needless compromises. It also gives you practical tips for choosing the fastest-possible combination of hardware and software for doing word processing.

Chapter 14 helps you choose the fastest-possible combination of hardware and software for doing database work, document management, or contact management. It tells you what software features you can reasonably expect to have if you insist on choosing the fastest-possible software. It also gives you valuable tips for optimizing the speed of hardware and software systems for database work, document management, and contact management.

Chapter 15 gives you hardware and software tips for assembling the fastest-possible combination of hardware and software for accounting and for analyzing data with spreadsheets. It tells you what software features you can expect to have if you insist on using the fastest-possible combination of hardware and software.

Chapter 16 tells you what combination of hardware and software to choose in order to get the fastest-possible system for handling images and sound, as well as what software features you can insist on.

Chapter 17 tells you how to select a high-speed combination of hardware and software for networking. Like earlier chapters, it tells you what software features you can have if you insist on choosing the fastest-possible combination of hardware and software.

Chapter 18 tells you how to apply similar selection standards to software for miscellaneous uses, such as GUI Communications and faxing.

Part 1

Health and safety-related issues

1

A quick look at health & safety issues

THIS book is intended for anyone who uses a video display terminal, whether you use a computer at home or at another place of work. It should also be extremely helpful to anyone who has management or supervisory responsibilities for the health and safety of computer-using workers.

Why this particular book at this particular time? Because, within the ever-expanding world of computer users there is a growing awareness of health problems associated with the use of personal computers and other video display workstations. And there is a growing willingness, on the part of employers and workers alike, both to prevent and to minimize such problems in the future. Some of the reasons for this growing awareness include the following:

➤ Persistent publicity about severe injuries and occupational disabilities that occur to workers who spend long hours at computer workstations.[1] For example, newspaper employees have been hit especially hard by injuries.

➤ Publicity about possible relationships between computer-intensive work and health issues such as spontaneous aborted pregnancies.

➤ The high rate of occupational illness, due to repetitive motions that exceed the design specification of human backs, necks, arms, and hands. These account for more than half of all occupational illnesses reported.

➤ Persistent attempts to pass mandatory municipal, state, and federal standards. California is in the process of adopting laws that will apply statewide to private as well as public employment. The federal Occupational Safety and Health Administration (OSHA) will have passed federal laws that will apply nationwide by the time this book hits the stores. And, industry-supported groups such as the American National Standards Institute (ANSI) and the American Society for Testing

1 "A Spreading Pain and Cries for Justice," The New York Times, June 5, 1994, pp. B3, B6.

and Materials (ASTM) are formulating standards that, though not law, could carry considerable weight in litigation.

➤ The medical and legal costs of office workers recovering under current laws strain the resources of the workers' compensation system and threaten its very viability, for both the physical injuries and their associated costs are quite significant.

All of this helps explain why experts in ergonomics (also called biotechnology) have finally been called in to provide solutions. In the current situation the science of ergonomics seeks to apply both biological and engineering data to a broad range of problems brought about by man's physical interactions with his newest machines. In that sense, throughout the remainder of this book any further references to "ergonomic seating" will mean seating that at least attempts to position the bodies of computer users comfortably and correctly, to maximize output while minimizing or even eliminating injury. Unfortunately, though ergonomics can help bring the needs of both man and machine together and can reconcile some of their differences, it can't cure a bad job after the fact by adding a few external accessories, such as an adjustable chair, wrist pads, or splints.

Preferably, at a much more fundamental level, computer-related jobs must be redesigned to bring certain kinds of work within the limits of human capability. But before designers can offer more functional designs they must know about much more than accessories to comprehend the true nature of the problems. They must understand how much and how little so-called "ergonomic" accessories can help, based on solid facts about how the body works and how it can break down in the office work setting.

These chapters will demonstrate how a basic knowledge of the critical ways in which human physiology relates to the workplace can help in analyzing an office workstation, and the office work pattern, for injury-causing potential.

In the past, many books and articles have been written about office ergonomics from the viewpoint of occupational medicine and biomechanics, describing the specific structures of muscles, tendons, bones, nerves, and circulation involved in the various problems.[2] Several good books have also been written by university professors, providing valid analyses of poor computer workstation design and including recommendations for better design.[3] You will also find published standards providing recommendations for VDT workstation design.[4]

Such information is valid but not very useful in an applied setting in which a manager must select and arrange the real components of an actual workstation. The texts usually provide line drawings of an idealized workstation, including an idealized person sitting bolt upright in an idealized "ergonomically correct" chair, at an idealized computer workstation in which all the ideal dimensions, in every conceivable direction, have been carefully calibrated. Unfortunately, no specific sources of components fitting the resulting requirements are mentioned.

Supervisors and workers in real life must evaluate and choose among real chairs and workstation components, none of which look like the drawings. And all may be touted as meeting ANSI/HFS standards.

The material in this book is based on almost two decades of experience in dealing with workstation problems as experienced by real individuals. We will provide valid information about real chairs. We will even examine a few of the most popular, giving you some basis for evaluating how various seating options may interact with workstation design, actual keyboards, supporting surfaces, and other paraphernalia.

2 A good example would be: M. Noidin, and V. H. Frankel, *Basic Biomechanics of the Musculoskeletal System, Second Edition*, Malvern, PA: Lem & Febiger, 1989.

3 A good example would be: Etienne Grandjean, *Ergonomics in Computerized Offices*, New York: Taylor & Francis, 1987.

4 "American National Standard for Human Factors Engineering at Visual Display Terminal Workstations," *ANSI/HFS 100*, Santa Monica, CA: Human Factors Society, 1988.

We will also describe some general issues related to computer work, such as health problems, workers' compensation for disabilities, cost savings, video monitor radiation, standardization, and government regulation. For example, re-engineering (automation) of computer-intensive work could well be one of the ways to reduce the health problems now associated with this work.[5]

We will also discuss some of the basic problems of lighting, noise, and visual distraction. We will suggest ways to provide necessary work surfaces in relatively small work areas, and the significant effects of these variables on the productivity of office workers. We will also offer names and contacts for information and assistance.

Finally, chapters on computer workstation standards and on worker's compensation will respond directly to supervisory and managerial concerns about controlling costs and liabilities while meeting the needs of workers.

5 The term VDT refers to video display terminal, which is often one of many connected to a central mainframe computer. The expressions "computer" and "computer workstation" will be used to refer to both a VDT and a personal computer with a video display monitor and a keyboard.

Ergonomic seating & how the body works

I F you look very far you will find a confusing proliferation of lists and drawings showing numerical specifications for ergonomic seating and workstation adjustments. These differ from one salesperson to the next and from one technical reference to the next. So, who do you believe? And what's so important about ergonomic chairs anyway?

This chapter will help you answer these questions. The important criteria for good ergonomic seating and workstation design become fairly obvious once you know a few basic facts about the remarkable structure of the human body.

In this and the next two chapters we will examine the odd curvature of the human spine and the tough "washers" of cartilage that separate and cushion spinal segments. We also consider the clever one-way valves in the fluid transport systems of the body. In lobster-pot fashion they permit particles such as blood cells, corpuscles, and bacteria to move only one way (usually up) through the system. An understanding of these factors alone should help the reader understand what ergonomic seating is about, and should lead to more confident consideration of seating alternatives.

The lumbar curve supports the weight of the upper body

The human spine has a natural double curvature in the rough form of a seahorse (see Fig. 2-1). Why this shape? It works for the seahorse because it helps him navigate and hide among the seaweed in the sea. For land-dwelling people, more likely reasons are those of balancing and supporting the weight of the upper body and head, and to provide extra flexibility and spring in the column as a whole. The spine must bend for this task, as your wrist must bend backward in holding a heavy weight in the palm of your hand. Also, two curves are required if the head is to be centered on the body. The upper curve (cervical, or neck) supports your head in the same way the lower curve (lumbar) down by your pelvis supports your upper body.

Figure 2-1

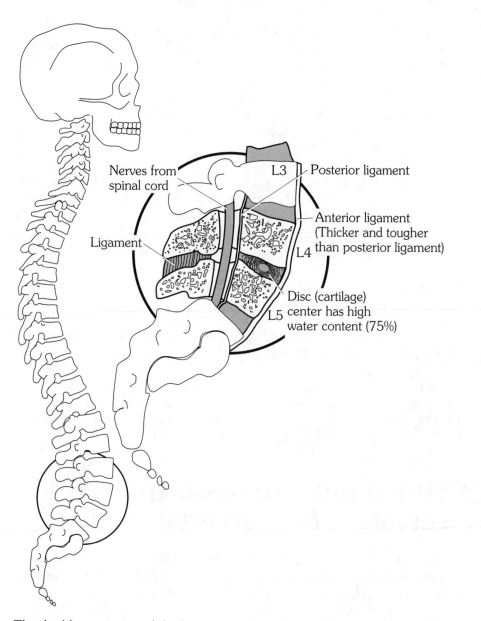

Nerves from spinal cord

L3

Posterior ligament

Anterior ligament
(Thicker and tougher
than posterior ligament)

Ligament

L4

Disc (cartilage)
center has high
water content (75%)

L5

The double curvature of the human spine, with an enlargement around the L4/L5 disc.

The term "lordosis" refers to the normal state of curvature in the lumbar and cervical sections of the spine. Some medical texts use the term to refer to excessive lordosis (swayback). Both uses are common.

The spine does not actually bend to form lordosis; rather the curves are built into the spine by the slight wedge shapes of the vertebrae, and by the slight wedge shapes of the angle between them as can be seen in Fig. 2-1.

The pressures under lumbar discs (e.g., L5) increase when bending over or sitting. When sitting? How can sitting increase pressure on discs? Is there no truth in the saying, "Sit down and take a load off"? True for the legs; not true for the spine. To understand how pressure increases with sitting, take a look at the lumbar discs L4/L5 in Fig. 2-1.

Discs are made of a tough material, like cartilage but layered like the plies of a radial tire, surrounding a mostly liquid center (see Fig. 4-1, p. 49). The discs compress and flex to allow spinal bending and turning. Thoracic (chest) vertebrae resist bending or turning because of their connection to the rib cage.

The discs get smaller during the day as fluid is squeezed out under pressure. Thus, one loses height during the day, which is gained back during sleep at night. In the weightlessness of space flight, astronauts gained as much as two inches in height (White 1990).

⇨ Sitting puts stress on spine curvature & intervertebral discs

The seated worker in Fig. 2-2 is a common sight. She is sitting in a slumped-forward posture, which has straightened her normal lordosis. This straightening, which puts strong pinching pressure on lumbar discs, is called "kyphosis." This is a very common posture during desk and keyboard work. In typical fashion the forward-leaning worker is not getting support from her chair back.

In a sitting position, hamstring muscles pull the bottom of the pelvis forward, reducing lordosis. Andersson (et al. 1979) found that lumbar

Figure 2-2

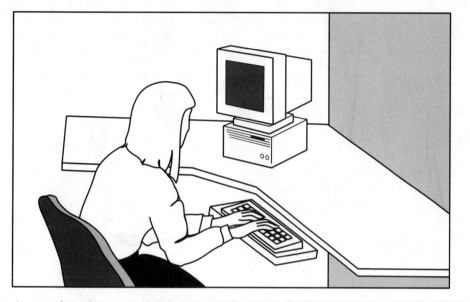

A seated worker in forward slumped (kyphosed) posture.

lordosis decreased by 38° when the subject moved from standing to unsupported sitting. This was the sum of a 28° pelvis tilt and a 10° flattening of lordosis around L4 and L5, as illustrated in Fig. 2-3. This kind of spinal distortion is increased even more when the seated person allows the pelvis to slide forward in the chair seat.

There are two kinds of slumping. In one, the person's upper back is bent away from the back of the chair as he leans forward to do his work. In the second, the pelvis moves away from the chair back as it slides forward on the chair seat. It is common to find both kinds of slumping at the same time in office workers.

In Fig. 2-2 sitting has increased compressive force at the front of the disc and has stretched the posterior ligament at the back of the disc. The disc has been pushed against the posterior ligament (Fig. 4-2, p. 50, also illustrates this). Both kinds of slumping increase this stress on spinal discs.

Figure 2-4 shows L3 disc pressures measured under standing and some sitting positions (Andersson et al. 1979, pp. 52–58). Most stressful was bending forward over work, creating an acute angle between spine and thigh.

Figure 2-3

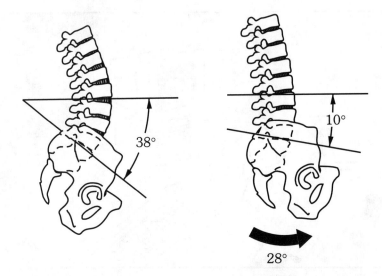

Pelvis tilt, when sitting.

Lumbar support from a chair back releases some stress, but only if it contacts the back. A properly designed chair seat that inhibits pelvic sliding can also lessen the stress of sitting somewhat. Arm support also reduces spinal stress.

The greatest spinal stress reduction comes from leaning backwards at least 110° into a lumbar-supporting chair back. This position is most relaxing for cervical as well as lumbar disc pressures. Arm support provides an additional reduction of pressure in this position.

Prolonged sitting wears and tears on discs, posterior ligaments, and muscles. The wear and tear is not often signaled by pain. Thus, seating habits and guidelines should be preventive, and the selection of sitting positions should be guided by knowledge as well as by pain reduction.

Seating design can minimize pelvis tilt & lumbar disc pressure

Given the importance of minimizing pelvis tilt and maintaining normal lordosis, a few well-known chairs advertised as "ergonomic" will be

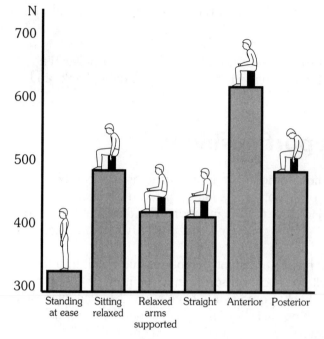

Figure 2-4

Lumbar disc pressure measurements (L3). The upper chart shows disk pressure while standing and seated with no arm support, while the lower shows the same for some seated postures. Note that 500N = approx. 112 lb. Adapted from Andersson, Murphy, Oertengren, and Nachemson, 1979

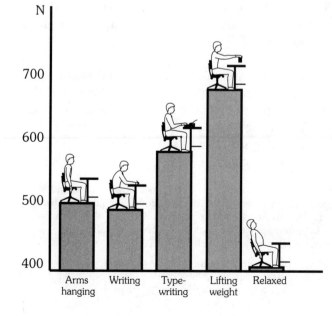

examined for characteristics that can reduce slumping, pelvis tilt, and disc pressure.

Several chair characteristics have the effect of reducing pelvis tilt: lumbar-support cushions, forward seat-pan tilt, a moving back, and others.

Lumbar-support cushions

Lumbar-support cushions range from loose cushions that can be strapped to the back of a chair, to padding, or to an air bladder built into the chair back. Tichauer (1978) mentioned studies that have shown workers wasting several hours per week keeping cushions in place.

A well-designed chair has an adjustable lumbar cushion built into the chair back, so that tall and short persons can move it up or down to fit into the small of their back. Some sitters have been observed increasing lumbar support by pushing their bottoms into the gap between the seat pan and the chair back. A well-designed chair will permit this.

The current voluntary standard for VDT workstation design, ANSI/HFS 100 (1988) pp. 59–60 of that document,[1] states that seating shall have a back rest with lumbar support on it, at a height 6 to 9 inches above the seat pan.

If we are correct in emphasizing the importance for good posture of preventing pelvis slumping, it becomes more important for the back support cushion to press against the back of the pelvis than to press into the lumbar arch.[2] Thus a back-support cushion positioned *below* the lumbar arch, and pushing against the back of the pelvis, should be more comfortable than a lumbar cushion.

1 *ANSI/HFS 100, 1988* refers to a set of recommendations put together by an industry-sponsored group, American National Standards Institute, together with the members of the professional group, the Human Factors and Ergonomics Society. Full publication information appears in the Bibliography at the back of this book; hereafter, this document will be referenced in the text as ANSI/HFS 100 (1988).

2 D. Zacharkow, a physical therapist, made this point in a physical therapy journal, *Physical Therapy Forum*, Sept. 10, 1990, pp. 2–5.

Given a need for pelvis support, the back-support cushion on a chair back should be lowerable to points lower than the 6-inch limit indicated by current ANSI/HFS standards. Lumbar or pelvis cushions or supports do little to support lordosis unless the sitter leans his pelvis against the back. Several methods used to encourage leaning against the chair back are included under the next three subheads below.

⇨ Pelvis pocket

Remember the wooden chairs you sat in when you were a kid? Remember how the back of the wood seat pan was dished out to help prevent sliding forward on the varnished surface into an uncomfortable scrunched-up slump? This slump-preventing pocket helped you sit up straight, back against the chair, by preventing pelvis tilting. The pelvis was captured in the pocket, and this helped delay kyphotic slumping. Also, many of these old chairs had slats in the back, curved in the lumbar area to provide additional support of lordosis. We would sit up straight for awhile but would eventually give in to the need for movement and slide back into a slump. The struggle would repeat itself throughout the sitting period.

Figure 2-5

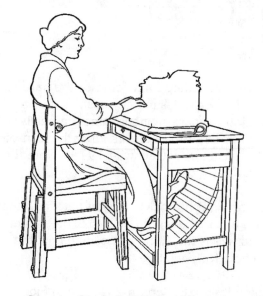

An adjustable chair with pelvis pocket (1919). From Remington Office Manual, Cited in Galloway, 1919

Stenographic desk with special foot rest.
This type of foot rest is designed to relieve fatigue.

Figure 2-6

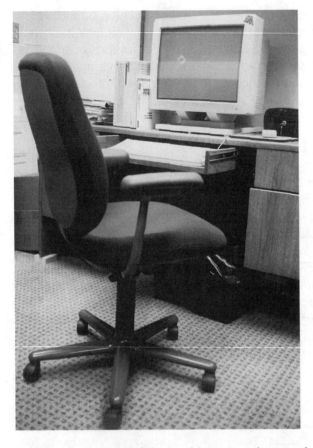

Herman-Miller Ergon (1) office chair. Herman-Miller

Foam seat cushions felt good because they took some of the hard seat-pan pressure off the two ischial tuberosities (butt bones). Unfortunately, with the evolution of foam seat cushions the pelvis pocket was generally covered up. Figure 2-5 shows an early, turn-of-the-century version of an adjustable chair (Galloway 1919). Note the pronounced pelvis pocket.

The Herman-Miller company brought the pelvis pocket back into foam seat cushions with the Ergon I chair, shown in Fig. 2-6. The pocket helps prevent pelvis tilting and keeps the spine pressed against the lumbar support in the chair back, for a while.

The most recent Herman-Miller design, the Ergon 2 (shown in Fig. 2-7), has largely lost the pelvis pocket. The pocket has been enlarged so

Figure 2-7

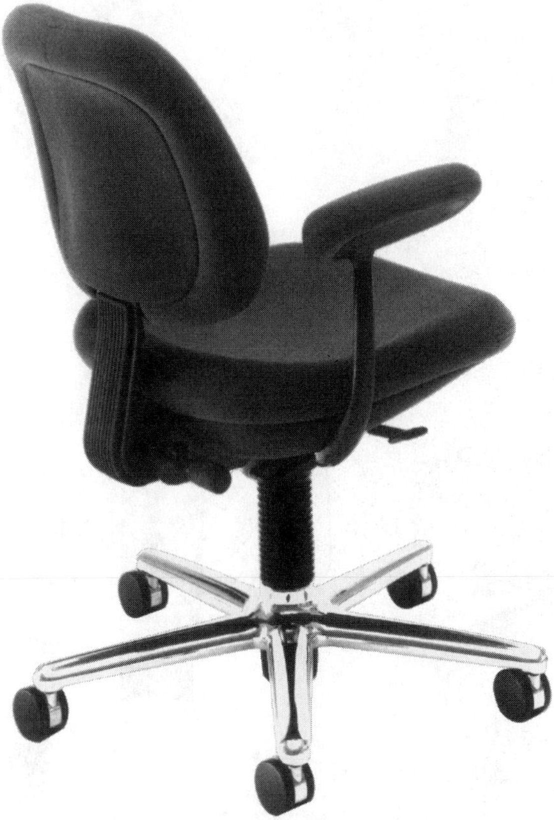

Herman-Miller Ergon (2) office chair. Herman-Miller

much that the front edge of the pocket, now being the front edge of the seat pan, puts some uncomfortable edge pressure in back of the knees. The need for movement eventually lends some sitters to slump in these chairs forward or backward just as in other chairs, as shown in Fig. 2-8.

A few words about slumping: It's not always bad for you. Forward slumping relaxes large postural muscles that must be tensed extra tight to hold a sitter in a static, upright, non-slumped posture. Large, strong muscles (erectors) use the back of the pelvis as an anchor to pull the spine into an upright position. They pull hard, back and down, on vertebrae and ribs, like guy wires raising a circus tent. Other muscles supporting the spine come from the abdominal group and from inside the thighs. They pull forward and down on the lumbar spine and ribs and, along with the erectors, help maintain spinal lordosis. Sitting relaxes these forward-originating guy wires, putting extra pressure on

Figure 2-8

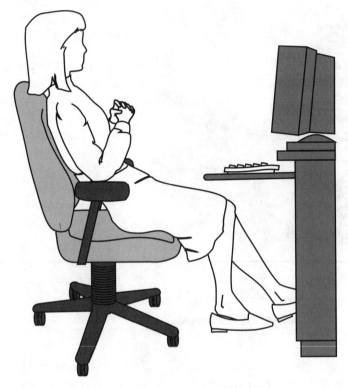

VDT worker leaning back in Ergon (1) chair.

the erectors, which now have to strain extra hard to maintain lordosis. Under the extra tension, and lacking the movement needed for normal muscle metabolism, the erectors soon fatigue and we tend to slump one way or the other. Brief episodes of forward slumping can also help provide some of the vertebral movement necessary for disc metabolism.

Although the Herman-Miller Company did not effectively address the need for backward leaning in the Ergon I and Ergon 2 designs, it must be commended for considering the primary role of preventing pelvis tilt and pelvic slumping for maintaining lordosis and sitter comfort, at least in its Ergon I chair. Many companies just put a lump of foam in the lumbar area of a straight chair back and say they provide an ergonomic (lordosis-supporting) chair. An *effective* lumbar-supporting chair will provide features for ensuring that the sitter *uses* that support, such as a pelvis pocket, an adjustable back angle, and an adjustable seat pan (see "Downward pan tilt" on following page).

⇨ Fabric

A rough woven fabric will help delay slumping out of the pelvis pocket. If your chair doesn't have a pelvis pocket (few do), slick coverings like vinyl, taut leather, or fine-woven polyesters will increase the amount of sliding, slumping, and eventual back pain. A loose weave will also help air circulation in the seat and prevent sweating.

⇨ Seat-pan length

If the seat pan is too long, short individuals will not be able to contact the lumbar support on the chair back. Taller individuals may want longer pans for more thigh support. There are only a few chair companies that provide length-adjustable seat pans (Discovery Seating Company is one) or backs that can be adjusted in-out (Bodybilt). The ANSI/HFS 100 (1988) voluntary standard recommends a seat depth between 15 and 17 inches, but it also suggests that the sitter's back should make contact with the lumbar area.

It is essential that chairs from several manufacturers be available in your office area, because some have larger pans than others. A variety of pan lengths meets the need for a variety of workers in the least expensive way.

⇨ Downward pan tilt

Next time you watch orchestral musicians playing notice the erect, lordotic, straight-back seated posture they maintain. They are most likely not leaning against their chair backs, at least not when they are playing. Notice the funny-looking chairs they are sitting on, with seat pans that are not level. They tilt *down*.

The slight down-sloping chair reduces pelvis tilt in the seated musician. Reducing pelvis tilt helps maintain lordosis. In addition to minimizing back pain, this position reduces slouching and slumping and so reduces pressure on the diaphragm and lungs, which must be unconstrained to permit expanding and contracting to their fullest during a physically demanding performance.

Figure 2-9

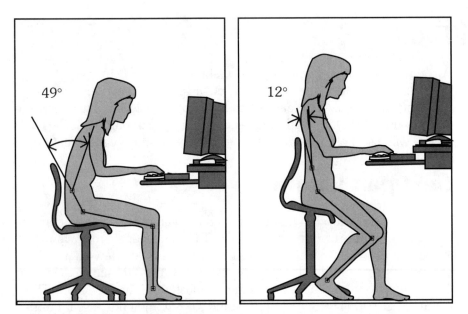

The effect of forward tilt on slumping (kyphosis). The left picture shows slumping posture, while the right shows the effect of forward tilt.

Figure 2-10

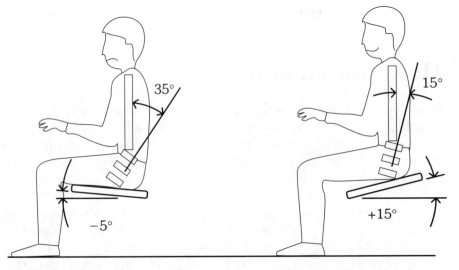

The right picture shows Mandel's conception of forward tilt effects on the lumbar spine.

Mandel (1981) has emphasized the point that downward tilt in a task chair can reduce pelvic tilt and the subsequent back pain that comes from both kinds of slumping. Figures 2-9 and 2-10 illustrate the effect of downward pan tilt and kyphotic slumping.

Several chair companies offer downward tilt. Steelcase provides downward tilt in its Criterion task chair. The logic of Mandel's reasoning for downward pan tilt is shown in the right panel of Fig. 2-9 and Fig. 2-10. The Bodybilt task chair (see Fig. 2-11) seems to provide the most effective downward tilt because of the slight saddle shape of its seat pan. The saddle shape reduces the sensation of tipping or sliding that may occur when a person first tries the down-tilt option. This sensation disappears with a bit of experience. Several of my clients use and appreciate this feature for computer and desk work.

Regarding downward pan tilt, ANSI/HFS 100 (1988) says simply that chairs with forward or backward tilting seat pans are acceptable. However, seats that tilt forward should use a fabric that prevents sliding.

Figure 2-11

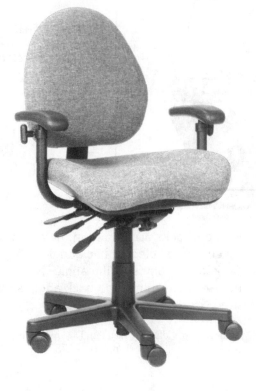

Bodybilt task chair.

23

Adjustable & dynamic backrest angle

A very effective way to encourage the sitter using the lumbar support is that of providing a chair back that can be pushed back to achieve the "relaxed" position depicted in Fig. 2-4. This position not only ensures using the lumbar support, but directly reduces the degree of pelvic tilt. In doing so, it greatly reduces pressure on lumbar discs. No wonder Grandjean, Hunting, and Pidermann found this position (see Fig. 2-12) preferred by most of the VDT workers in their 1983 study.[3]

Figure 2-12

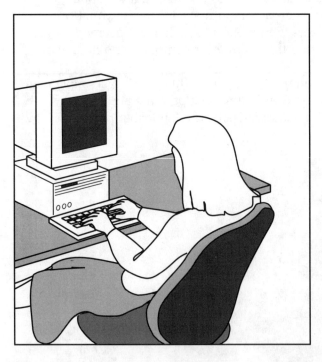

Typical seated posture at a video display workstation.

Two types of angle-adjustable chair backs are common, in which the angle-settable back can be locked into a selected back angle. The "dynamic" chair back is not locked into any specific angle. Rather, the back is tension-loaded and the user determines the back angle simply by leaning back as far as desired, or to a limit.

3 E. Grandjean, W. Hunting, and M. Pidermann, "VDT Workstation Design: Preferred Settings and Their Effects," *Human Factors*, 25(2), 1983, pp. 161–175.

The Bodybilt chair has an angle-settable back, which is used by many of my CAD worker clients. Harter also has an angle-settable back in their Anthro model task chair.

A dynamic back may turn out to be the most popular approach to angle adjustment since it is automatic; you just lean back. A dynamic back that is also angle-settable should appear within the next two years. More will be said about dynamic back support in Chapter 6, which deals with postural fixity and the importance of movement.

Two dynamic back chairs are shown below and on following page—the Sensor by Steelcase (Fig. 2-13) and the Comforto by Haworth (Fig. 2-14).

Figure 2-13

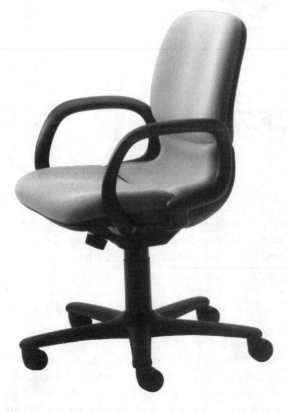

Common video display workstation chair: the Steelcase Sensor. Steelcase

Figure 2-14

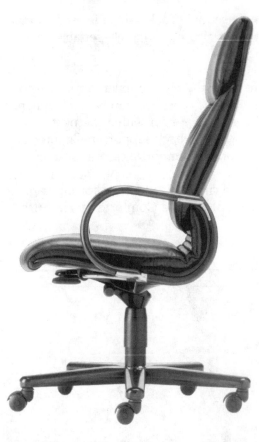

Common video display workstation chair: the Haworth Comforto. Haworth

Both of these chairs allow one to simply lean back and take some weight off the spinal discs and muscles while answering the phone, talking to a colleague or guest, keyboarding, or just thinking. They are nice-looking chairs, both designed by famous stylists; Sensor by Wolfgang Mueller-Deisig, Comforto by Simon Desanto.

The manager version of Comforto is shown for two reasons. First, to show that a functional feature (for example, prominent lumbar support) can also be a positive design feature. This particular lumbar support is not adjustable, but it should fit quite a few sitters. Second, to show a manager/executive chair that is quite functional. Executive and manager chairs are often overstuffed, thronelike, and not suitable as working chairs. The task (worker) version of Comforto has a shorter back but the same functions. Knoll has a chair, the 700 Series, with a similar appearance.

Let us examine both the Sensor and Comforto chairs more closely. A pelvis pocket would help prevent pelvic slumping in the Comforto, especially on taut leather and polyester fabric options. The dynamic back, which yields when the sitter leans back, does a good job of preventing upper body slump in both chairs. The prominent lumbar support does not ride up on the spine to any significant extent when the sitter leans back in the Comforto. If you test both chairs you will find the dynamic action of the Sensor a bit more responsive than that of Comforto to tension adjustment. For this reason Sensor may be easier for small, light persons to use. However, since Comforto has more prominent lumbar support, located relatively low, leaning back in Comforto should take more pressure off intervertebral discs than doing the same thing in Sensor.

⇨ Arms

Now look at the arms on these chairs. The arms are narrow and hard. The elbow wobble and slide on these is similar to what you get on the arms between economy-class airline seats. You cannot make a significant impression when you push your thumb into them. For this reason, these chairs cannot be recommended for anyone who spends more than an hour a day at a keyboard. The arms are not adjustable so they may just get in the way of some users, causing some to hunch their shoulders and others to work with no forearm support.

Arm supports should be designed as forearm supports in task chairs, because they should not press against the elbows, where important nerves run around the elbow close to the skin.

The Sensor Line now presents adjustability options for arms and lumbar support, at extra cost. The basic, bare-bones Sensor model, with hard, narrow arms and negligible, nonadjustable lumbar support has been featured here because the bare-bones model of any chair line is the one that keyboarders and other employees tend to get stuck with. The reason for that is individual workers seldom have any say in the selection of their seating. The selection is usually made by an

27

office manager, administrative officer, or facilities procurement personnel, with the help of interior decorators and a budget manager. Sometimes an architect does the choosing. The result is overriding attention to appearance, uniformity, and cost factors (including initial price, sturdiness, and availability) with inadequate or unskilled attention to the ergonomic needs of actual employees.

Because price is related to quality, and the average life of a well-built chair extends over ten years, a common situation is an occupational army of these indestructible dinosaurs hanging around the office for ages, preventing improvement in the available seating. Workers park their old chairs out in the halls, hoping they will disappear. A storage area with any extra space soon gets filled up with them. Areas become "storage depots" by harboring these fugitives. You can find them hiding under stairwells. A lot of those wide, Pollack-styled chairs with hard plastic arms and 19- by 21-inch seat pans collect in such places. At the same time, as a capital investment, a chair has outlived its usefulness as a tax credit after only five years.

Chair designs are slowly improving, but until they achieve a general state of adequacy, which is many years away, and more ergonomic and worker input enters into the selection process, physical sturdiness will be of doubtful virtue. There are less expensive chairs with the same features as major brands. Globe furniture[4] is one example of a low-cost supplier of chairs with some ergonomic features. The warranty and service agreement may be less favorable than that of the more highly advertised brands, but such may be the cost-effective way to go for now.

ANSI/HFS 100 (1988) does not address angle-adjusted backs, but it does specify chairs that allow leaning back at back angles greater than 105°, with back rests sufficiently high to support the upper trunk, head, and neck.

The head support seems generally unnecessary, but such chairs are useful to people with cervical damage who have difficulty holding their heads up. At this time most angle-adjustable task chairs do not have adequate trunk-supporting back height.

4 Globe Business Furniture (Synergy Line), 90 Volunteer Drive, Hendersonville, TN 37075.

Two last points about angle-adjustable backs. First, as the back-pan angle opens up the lumbar support must not ride up, or move to a higher point on the spine to an uncomfortable extent. Second, the front edge of the seat pan must not press up uncomfortably on the user's thighs or lift his feet off the floor. These refinements can be achieved by designs that either move the pivot forward on the pan or have the pan and back move at different rates (Fig. 2-15).

Figure 2-15

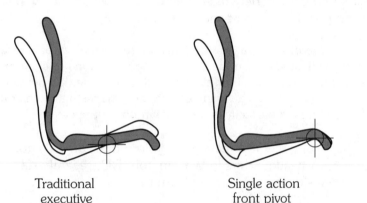

Traditional
executive

Single action
front pivot

Seat-pan movements, showing the front pivot
movement that minimizes pressure behind the knees.

One additional factor to consider in evaluating a chair back is the *width* of the back. All modern office chairs are of the swivel-type that you can spin around. This makes it easy to turn left or right and reach for the phone or the printer. However, if you sit close to your desk or keyboard it may be inconvenient to turn your chair left or right. A narrow chair back (Bodybilt, Fig. 2-11) may make it easier for you to turn and reach.

⇨ One chair does not fit all

One thing that I've learned in seventeen years of watching sitters is that one chair model, and not even one chair line, can meet the variety of seating needs for any group of more than two or three people. One must provide several ergonomically qualified, but different, alternatives for each worker to select from. Significant arm options should be present for worker tryout. When you talk to each worker, and have them write their evaluations after they try each chair for several days, you will be surprised at the variety of valid individual differences in seating needs. It is like buying shoes. Only the individual wearer can provide information relevant to fit, and one style and size is not going to fit very many people. These sentiments agree with those expressed in a very readable publication of the American Medical Association[5] dealing with back care. After a beautiful presentation of cases illustrating how the variety of seating needs must be met with a variety of seating possibilities, on pages 136–137 it says:

> . . . all too often chairs are designed more for their appearance than for their effect on the body. Yet no single type of chair or sitting position is ideal for everyone all of the time. We human beings come in such a variety of sizes and shapes that a chair that fits one person perfectly may be all wrong for the next . . .

Given this strong medical recommendation, one can only guess why the new AMA headquarters in Washington, DC, recently standardized on a single task chair (Anthro by Harter).

There are significant differences between males and females in factors that relate directly to appropriate seating. For example, females tend to have more natural lordosis than males, and their upper body size, weight, and musculature is less in relation to lower body size and weight. The female spine is centered over a point relatively closer to the back of the pelvis than is the case for males. This enables a woman to stand, back against a wall, bend over, and pick up a chair, a feat men cannot duplicate without falling forward. Male-female differences are yet another reason why a single chair type and model will not fit all of your office workers.

Harter has a narrow, short-pan version of their Anthro chair, which may be more suitable for females, on average, than their standard model. Also, the relatively short seat pan of Comforto may make this task chair suitable for many women.

Large, wide workers have trouble locating chairs that fit. Bodybilt has a large-size version of its task chair that can fill this need.

5 M. Steinmann, *The American Medical Association Guide to Back Care*, New York: Random House, 1989.

Research by Tichauer (1973) has shown workers wasting an average of 3.5 hours per week dealing with poor seating. The amount of wasted time can be much greater than this for some individuals. It will pay to deal with seating problems on an individual basis.

⇨ Standing and sit-stand seating

Chair design can help reduce the degree of pelvic tilt when users are sitting, but more drastic measures may be necessary for computer workers, or any other workers, who sit a good portion of the day. In the past, standing has been a postural option for desk work. Tall, slanted, standing worktables used by architects, draftsmen, and engineers were common not so long ago. Figures 2-16 and 2-17 show a 1918 version for a stenographer (Galloway 1919).

Figure 2-16

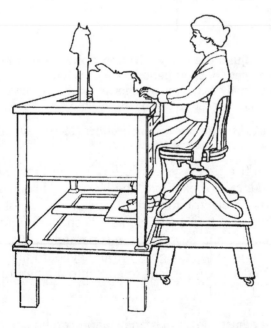

Adjustable desk - Stenographer sitting
The desk and chair are placed on platforms so that the operator can work either in a sitting or standing posture, as she prefers.

Sit-Stand workstation for a stenographer (1919)—sitting.

31

Figure 2-17

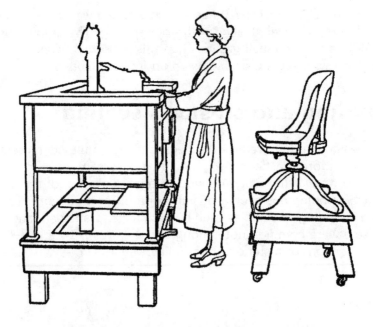

Adjustable desk - Stenographer standing
To work standing for short periods of time is found to relieve fatigue.
With chair and desk raised, as shown above, the change from a
sitting posture can be made almost instantly.

Sit-Stand workstation for a stenographer (1919)—standing.

Some modern office panel systems offer an adjustable work surface
that allows standing. For example, the Herman Miller Ethospace
System provides an electric-motorized version. A free-standing version
offered by Human Factors Technologies[6] is shown in Fig. 2-13. The
surfaces for monitor and keyboard are separately adjustable. The
keyboard surface is wide enough for both keyboard and mouse, and
there is room underneath for legs to stretch out when the user wants
to lean back (Fig. 2-18).

An inexpensive adjustable sit-or-stand station can be constructed by
obtaining a motorized drafting table at a used office furnishings store.
They are plentiful in some areas now that designers and engineers do
their work sitting at CAD video stations. Have the large table surface

6 SIS Human Factor Technologies, Inc., 55 Harvey Road, Londonderry, NH 03053.

Figure 2-18

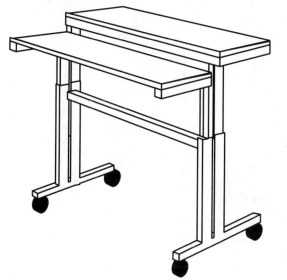

Bi-level work table.

sawed off to fit your needs, then just push the pedal to raise the surface enough to permit standing until your back and neck feel better. The static, unmoving nature of standing will lead to leg muscle fatigue, but the change of posture from sitting to standing is important for a healthy back. Movement while standing, such as putting one foot up on a foot rest (analogous to a bar rail) can delay the onset of standing fatigue.

A sit-stand posture is fairly common in industrial work settings. This posture, depicted on the following page, permits the lordosis that is characteristic of standing, along with a fairly open, untilted pelvis, and removes some of the static weight from leg muscles. This posture, which is maintainable longer than standing, requires a seat pan design that differs from traditional chair pan design (Fig. 2-19).

Many chair companies offer chairs that can be adjusted high enough for sit-standing, but the seat pan does not tilt down. Herman-Miller and Harter are two companies that offer such nice tall chairs (i.e., stools). Steelcase, Herman-Miller, and Haworth, among others, are able to provide sit-stand seating, but the seat shapes still need work.

In the future, a chair will be designed that can support comfortable sit-standing, as well as sitting, at office work. When this happens, sit-

Figure 2-19

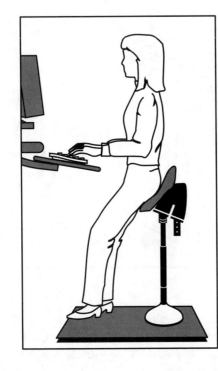

Sit-Stand VDT seating.

standing may become the posture of choice. It will certainly be harder to nod off in this position.

Patten has looked at the sit-stand seats offered by many companies, foreign and domestic. The Bio-Fit,[7] Protilt One (Fig. 2-14), and Ergostand, by Work-Rite,[8] seem to have a seat-pan design suited to sit-standing. Some sit-stand pads are built like bicycle saddle seats. You don't want casters or wheels on a sit-stand for obvious reasons. You could end up sitting on the floor.

The only ANSI/HFS 100 (1988) item related to standing or sit-standing is the discussion of seat height (pp. 52–53). A seat-height adjustability range of 16 to 20.5 inches is recommended.

Twenty inches is not nearly high enough for sit-standing. Apparently, writers of the current standard did not envision office workstation

7 Bio-Fit, P. O. Box 109, Waterville, OH 43566.

8 Work-Rite, 444 Saratoga Ave., #21-H, Santa Clara, CA 95050.

postures other than sitting, but that should not stop you from trying them out. Such experimentation for problem cases, or for prevention studies, will certainly help promote worker health.

A therapeutic chair for severe back pain sufferers

Discussion of chair design so far has emphasized factors that reduce pelvic tilt, as one way of minimizing the great pressure that sitting puts on lumbar discs. The elimination of gravity works even better, but requires special clothing and a space shuttle. We can dream of other possibilities: a cushion of forced air, or water from Salt Lake, perhaps. Actually, something like this has been developed. A small company, Spinal Designs,[9] has developed a sitting device that gently holds the sitter around the bottom of the rib cage. This mild, gravity traction reduces disc pressure by adjustable amounts. It is to be used three or four 10-minute periods per day, at home or office, by persons with back pain problems. It appears that these brief periods of disc-pressure relief can permit near-normal functioning during the rest of the day, and reduce the frequency of disabling episodes. The device is used under medical supervision.

Anything you can do to relieve back stress at home should help you get through the work day. One common source of back strain is a swayback mattress, that leads to lumbar kyphosis or side stress on lumbar discs and muscles. You wake up with a painful or stiff back. Ergonomic mattresses that can actually help have been developed. They are firm to prevent sway, but have enough pillowed padding on top of the firmness to provide body curvature support. A brand that works for me is Spring-Air Back Supporter Royale, Extra Firm. It was discovered fortuitously at a Sears warehouse sale. It has a label saying that it has the endorsement of a staff of orthopedic surgeons.

Have you ever wondered what possession you would try to save first if your house started to burn down?

9 Spinal Designs International, 2800 Chicago Ave. S., Suite 300, Minneapolis, MN 55407.

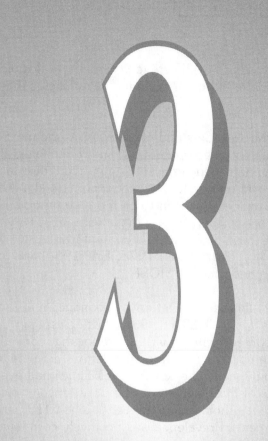

Seating & upper extremity pain

T HE cervical portion of the spine is even more flexible than the lumbar segment, although not quite as mobile as that of Linda Blair in *The Exorcist*.

Muscle tension in the shoulders and neck region is the most frequent health complaint of computer operators (Sauter, Schliefer, and Knutson 1991), and damaged cervical vertebrae and discs are common in adults. Huntington (et al. 1981) found tendon/muscle pain in the neck, shoulder, and arm to be more common among data entry and typing workers than among those with more varied office jobs. Prevalence of these problems in a computer-intensive workplace is indicated by surveys (Harris et al. 1978; Brill 1984) and in recent hazard evaluations conducted by NIOSH.

The most recently published evaluation was conducted at the offices of the *Los Angeles Times* (HETA 1993). Most newspaper employees use computers to some extent for writing, reporting, copyediting, entering advertising copy, accounting, circulation, news database access, and electronic mail. The Los Angeles Times had over 7500 workers at the time of this evaluation. The prevalence of disorders was neck (26 percent), shoulder (17 percent), elbow (10 percent), hand/wrist (22 percent). Prevalence was positively correlated with factors such as amount of time spent on the keyboard, amount of time spent working under deadlines, gender, and reports that one's section supervisor or manager was not concerned with worker health.

⇨ How seating affects cumulative trauma of the upper extremities

⇨ Head-neck angle

Chaffin (1973) looked at the relation between a sitter's head/neck angle and fatigue in neck-area muscles. He concluded that the head/neck angle (head hanging down) should not be greater than 20–30 degrees from horizontal for more than a few minutes. Head/neck angle is not to be confused with line of sight. The latter can be 15 degrees above or below the head/neck angle without discomfort.

⇨ A dynamic back support promotes posture variation

Grandjean (et al. 1983) used adjustable chairs and video monitors and found that 90 percent of the workers in this study preferred leaning back, behind vertical. He also found that, when leaning back, the leaner's preferred line of sight was about 10 degrees below horizontal. That fairly high viewing angle is automatically achieved without much monitor height adjustment, as one leans back behind vertical into the back-relaxed posture. The monitor can be tilted up or down and the keyboard can be lowered some to accommodate the new viewing angle. Thus a tiltable monitor is important for back and arm health.

ANSI/HFS 100 (1988) covers viewing angle while discussing height of the support surface. The discussion offers little specific guidance, stating that the appropriate height depends on seating design and user preference. It recommends that computer height should provide a line of sight between horizontal and 60 degrees below horizontal. Monitor height and tilt adjustability will help meet individual viewing angle preferences.

⇨ Headache

Tense, static muscles cut off their own blood flow. The resulting lack of oxygen and buildup of lactic acid cause fatigue and pain in these muscles. That is why long periods of muscle tension in the neck and upper back, used to maintain a given head/neck angle, can lead to headache as well as discomfort and muscle pain. Thus, changing your sitting posture frequently during the day can reduce the frequency of headache as well as neck and upper-back discomfort.

Many of us wake up in the morning with a sore neck. Presumably, preventing this would promote getting through a day at the office without neck or upper-back pain. One frequently sees ads for a cervical pillow to prevent morning neck stiffness. It supports the neck during sleep.

Figure 3-1

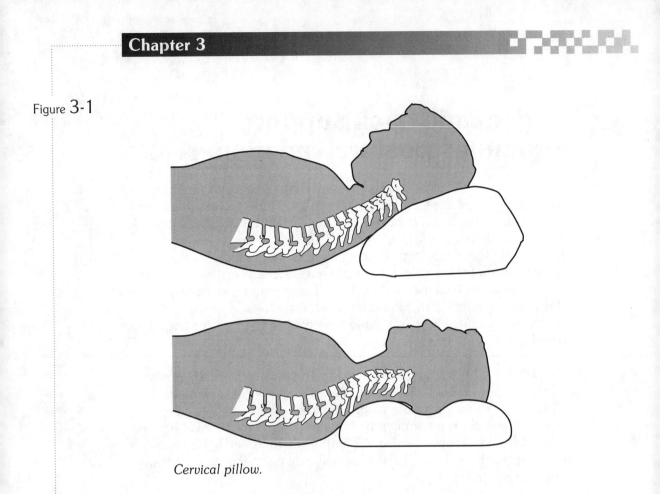

Cervical pillow.

This author (Patten) tried a cervical pillow with some success, but has found that stuffing enough of a normal pillow under the neck to support cervical lordosis has been just as effective. Give it a try (Fig. 3-1).

Arm rests

Neck, upper-back, and shoulder pain is often experienced by workers who hold their arms up while using the keyboard. One of the BOSTI Survey findings in 1984 concerned the arm and shoulder pain experienced by workers who did not have arm rests on their chairs (Brill 1984). This stress can be reduced by using comfortable, padded arm rests, adjustable to a correct height. Figure 2-4, in Chapter 2 (p. 15), shows how arm support can reduce spinal disc pressure. Arm supports also reduce static muscle tension, fatigue, and discomfort on neck, back, and shoulder muscles.

Chair arms that are too high can cause pain in one's neck, upper back, and shoulders, from prolonged static shoulder hunching. Figure 3-2 was drawn from a photograph of a colleague who hunched a lot because she used her desk top for arm support. She reported neck and shoulder pain, and sore elbows.

Figure 3-2

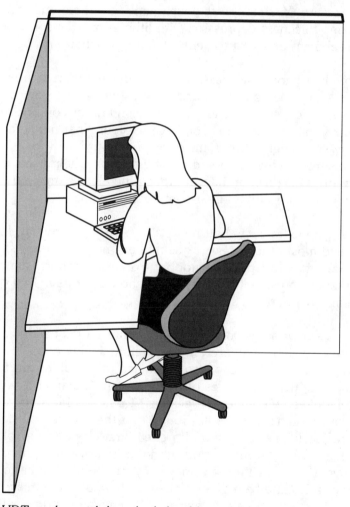

VDT worker with hunched shoulders and arms.

How can you tell if chair arms are large enough and have enough padding? You can do it in a practical way, by trying the chair a day or two, watching others use it, and by using a rule of thumb.

Do elbows wobble or slide when leaning on the arm? Herman Miller Ergon arms are soft enough so that elbows don't wobble or slide under pressure. You can press your thumb into them and create a near thumb-thickness depression with little effort. Sensor, Comforto, and Harter arms are hard to dent, as are most chair arms.

Cases of ulnar-nerve compression occur now and then with hard, small arms. This large nerve to the hand runs just under the skin, close to the elbow, which leaves it vulnerable to being hit or compressed. If you've hit your "funny bone" you have hit your ulnar nerve, and you also know the general symptoms of nerve compression: pain, tingling, lack of control, and weakness (dropping things). Chair arms that support forearms only, and do not touch the elbows, may turn out to be the best for preventing ulnar-compression pain.

The basic, no-extra-cost chair models of Sensor, Comforto, Harter, Ergon, and most others, have arms that are not height-adjustable and are not designed for forearm support. Forearm support is important for workers who use a keyboard several hours per day. Two options for forearm support are shown in Fig. 3-3.

Figure 3-3 shows a Bodybilt chair with "Minnesota" padded arms. These are adjustable and are long enough and wide enough to support forearms. They can also be angled (pivoted) inward to accommodate the arm angles of workers using a standard keyboard. Unfortunately they contact the elbows. A pair of Finnish clinical studies of swiveling arm cradles found that they decreased strain in the upper back muscles and the forehead muscles often involved in headaches.[1] The bottom portion of Fig. 3-3 shows forearm cradles that swivel to move with the arms. They can be used in either an upright or a leaning-back seated posture. It would be a mistake to get cradles that attach to a desk, because they would restrict seated posture and force upper-body slumping.

1 Cited in S. B. Leavitt, *Casualties at the Office*, Glenview, IL: Leavitt Medical Communications, 1994, p. 21.

Figure 3-3

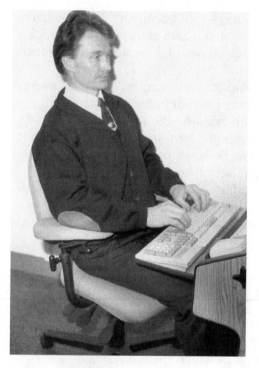

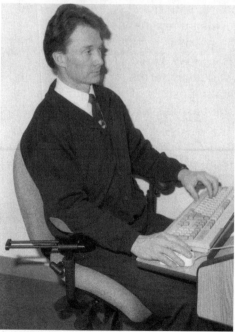

Bodybilt angle-adjustable chair arms. (a) Minnesota-type forearm support. (b) Cradle-type forearm support. Bodybilt Co.

The only thing ANSI/100 (1988) says about armrests is that, when they are provided, the distance between them shall be at least 18.2 inches. Most workers will need more than 14.2 inches between arms.

The next logical step to more complete arm support would be one of attaching the keyboard to the arms. The left half of the keyboard would be connected to the left arm rest and the right half of the keyboard would be attached to the right arm. In fact an adaptation similar to this is now available (Fig. 3-4).[2] This is potentially a very significant development for a number of reasons. First, it removes ulnar (outward) deviation and bending of wrists that is prevalent with standard keyboards. And second, it allows keyboarding from either a leaning-back or a sitting-up posture. Why is this important? There are several reasons.

It is a very interesting and promising development because removing the keyboard from the desk, or other fixed forward surface, and putting it on the chair eliminates the requirement for the worker to bend forward to the keying task. It allows a significant healthy break away from the customary slumped keyboard-working posture. The customary slumped posture is one in which the worker is bent forward, head bent over the keyboard, with hunched shoulders and tensed, fixated arms holding forearms up and hands over the keyboard. Neither the back nor the pelvis is resting against the chair back (see Fig. 3-2, p. 41). Muscles and vertebrae of the neck area strain to hold the head, hunched shoulders, arms, and hands rigidly suspend over the keyboard. The static posture of the arms, close to the body, can put pressure on blood vessels and nerves that pass from the chest along the undersides of the arms. The pain and disability from prolonged constriction of blood flow and nerve conduction in this area is a CTD (Cumulative Trauma Disorder) known as thoracic outlet syndrome.

In Chapter 5, another CTD known as carpal tunnel syndrome will be described as the numbness, pain, and disability that comes from nerve compression related to excessive wear and tear on tendons that control finger movement. The swelling from tendon friction puts disabling

2 Floating Arms Keyboard, Workplace Designs, Inc., 301–311 South Main Street, Stillwater, MN 55082. Phone/Fax: 612-439-4474

Figure 3-4

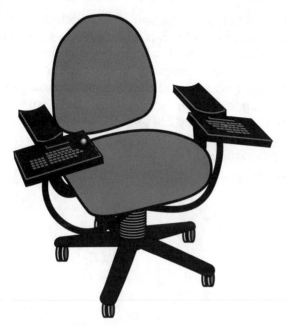

The "Floating Arms" Keyboard.

pressure on sensory nerves and muscle-control nerves in the wrist and hand. A variety of pain and disability syndromes, tendonitis, and other "-itises" and so-called "disease" conditions are associated with each other and tend to occur in the same individual at different times, or at the same time.

Notice how the "floating" keyboards are tilted in Fig. 3-4. The tilt is adjustable, and this seems to be the angle preferred by users. Thus, a neutral (most comfortable) wrist position is one that is tilted up a bit.

⇨ Summary

Seating that does not allow the worker to lean back beyond vertical while working produces a harmful slumped-forward, shoulders-hunched, upper-body posture. This posture puts excessive pressure on both the lower and the upper spine, and on the muscles that support the head, the arms, and the hands. This pressure leads to headache from muscle tension and blood-flow constriction; and the shoulder hunching constricts nerve and blood conduction from the chest through the thoracic outlet to arms and hands (see Zacharkow, 1994). Attempts to prop the slumping upper body with the elbows and forearms puts damaging pressure on nerves running around the elbows. These consequences of poor seated posture and slumping are associated with CTD of the upper extremities as well as back pain and spinal damage. Thus, poor seating really does set the stage for CTD.

The discussion of CTD will continue in Chapter 5 after we explain in Chapter 4 why one should sit as little as possible.

4

Postural fixity & the importance of activity

CHAPTER 4

THE unchanging, rigid nature of computer-worker posture is hard not to notice. It is recognized as a major problem of computer-intensive work. "In VDT work the lack of physical activity is probably more marked than in any other modern tasks" (Kilbom 1987). A recent Ergonomic Society feature lecture dealt specifically with this problem (Grieco 1986).

In production-oriented computer work the head, trunk, arms, and hands are kept in position over certain "home" keys for maximum input speed. The head is fixed in position for reading the input document, as well as focusing on small, fuzzy, video characters with a minimum of search time.

Lacking knowledge of human physiology, most people are prone to think that sitting is non-stressful and that sitting straight and still is good, healthful posture. Teachers and employers sometimes regard behaviors that deviate from this as misbehavior. In a recent case, a teacher chained a student to the back of his chair to make him sit up straight.[1]

But on the contrary, the general message of this chapter is that sedentary, fixed-position work is unhealthy. Sitting at a computer terminal for hours wears on muscle, bone, and blood circulation in ways that may surprise you. A few basic facts of physiology will show the remarkable manner in which the human body is designed for movement, and the destructive consequences of inactivity and postural rigidity. Movement will be related to intervertebral discs, blood circulation, intestinal function, the lymphatic system, and bone strength.

⇨ Intervertebral discs: body movement is the metabolic pump

It is an odd but true fact that adult intervertebral discs have no blood supply. Nutrients are pulled into the discs, and their waste products expunged, by the squishing and squeezing forces of adjacent

---

1 "Chained to His Desk," Minneapolis *Star Tribune*, July 12, 1994, p. 1B.

48

vertebrae during body movement. Like sponges they give up metabolic waste when squeezed between vertebrae, and soak up nutrients upon expansion when pressure is removed (Hansson 1986).

Lack of frequent body movement can lead to disc degeneration from deficiencies in oxygen and nutrients. The damaged disc is prone to further tearing from strong pinching forces that accompany slumped postures (Fig. 4-1).

Figure 4-1

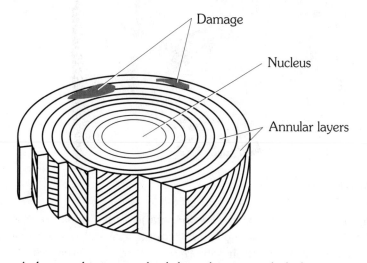

Damage

Nucleus

Annular layers

A damaged intervertebral disc, showing radial plies.

Most people think they do not have back problems unless there is back pain. The story is not that simple. Disc pressure, pinching, tearing, and other damage do not cause pain directly, because discs have little innervation and do not sense pain. This is unfortunate because disc pain could lead us to seek a healthier posture and thus prevent irreversible disc damage.

Repeated disc pinching from poor posture (sitting, lifting, twisting) can eventually lead to severe pain when a disc herniates, or breaks through the posterior ligament, as illustrated in Fig. 4-2.

Strong pain extending down the leg, called sciatica, is commonly attributed to lumbar disc herniation and compression of the nearby sciatic nerve. Small herniations, or protrusions, may be the ones that

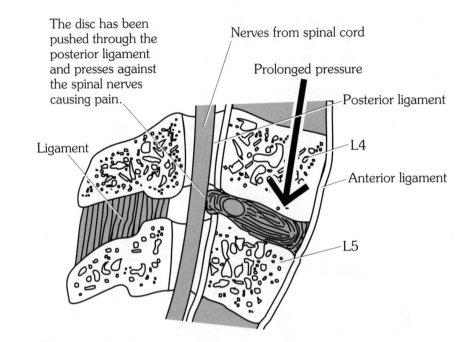

Figure 4-2

The disc has been pushed through the posterior ligament and presses against the spinal nerves causing pain.

Nerves from spinal cord

Prolonged pressure

Posterior ligament

Ligament

L4

Anterior ligament

L5

Herniated disc.

cause pain, while large, sustained herniation may cause numbness along with pain. J. L. Kelsey (1975) found that people who sat half or more of the time on their jobs had a 60 to 70 percent greater risk of herniating a disc than those who did not sit that much.

Muscles and blood vessels are richly innervated and do give us some warning of awkward or rigid posture when they report fatigue and pain. Khalil (et al. 1993) suggests that most low back pain is myofascial pain, due to tearing and inflammation of muscle and fascia (membrane that covers muscle) in the vicinity of lumbar vertebrae. Multiple trigger, or sensitive, points for pain and stiffness are symptomatic of this condition. Prolonged postural fixity and inactivity can put these kinds of pressures on lumbar muscles.

Lumbar muscle pain can also be caused when the tense, fixated muscle cuts off its own blood supply. The lack of oxygen and accumulation of lactic acid and metabolic waste stimulate pain receptors in the blood vessels and muscle (Khalil et al. 1993).

Pain in the neck, shoulder, and upper back can also be caused by the fixated posture common to computer work, especially if the worker's arms or back are unsupported, or if his shoulders are hunched. Myofasic and ischemic (reduced blood supply) pain are among the mechanisms for these cervical and thoracic pains.

If we pay attention to our initial feelings of back discomfort and pain, which come from oxygen-starved muscles, and this leads us to change posture and increase movement, we may very well prevent myofascial inflammation or disc damage. Unfortunately, people have a capacity to endure discomfort and pain and often think they have a duty to do so.

Blood circulation, body movement, & the venous pump

Prolonged inactivity leads surprisingly to *elevation* in blood pressure and heart rate (Sandler and Vernikos 1986) and to various disorders associated with blood pooling and clotting, such as phlebitis and thrombosis (citations in Winkel 1987). Phlebitis, which was President Nixon's disease, is a blood-clotting condition and is a frequent complication of varicose veins that is thought to be caused by blood pooling in veins (Baron 1979). It tends to flare up after long periods of sitting. Deep vein thrombosis (DVT), the clinical term for blood clot formation in the legs, can lead to serious pulmonary embolism if the DVT clot moves from leg to lungs and lodges in a major lung artery. DVT can occur after as little as three hours of inactive sitting. This has occurred on airplanes during cross-country and international flights. Articles in newspapers (*Star Tribune* 1988) and magazines (King 1993) have dubbed these cases, reported in the British medical journal *Lancet*, as "economy class syndrome" because economy class seating is more restrictive of activity than first class seating.

The pragmatic manager or worker will likely view these assertions with a skeptical eye, as possible exaggeration or alarmism, unless he or she has had personal experience with the problems described. But once the "mechanics" of the venous pump and blood clotting are understood it is easy to see how inactivity, and sitting, can produce such circulatory problems. The venous pump is illustrated in Fig. 4-3.

51

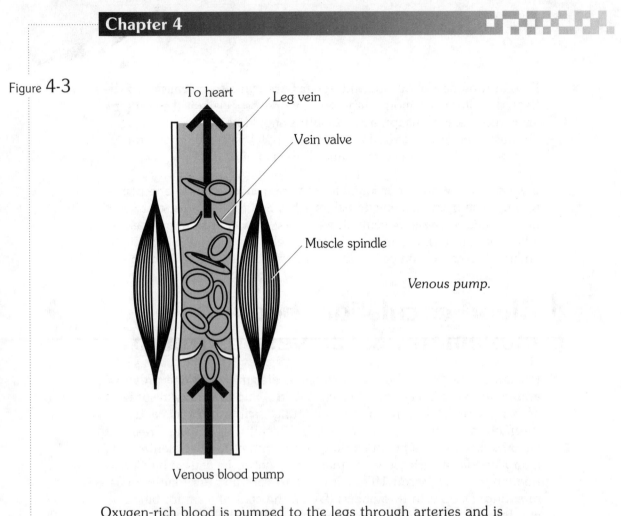

Figure 4-3

To heart

Leg vein

Vein valve

Muscle spindle

Venous pump.

Venous blood pump

Oxygen-rich blood is pumped to the legs through arteries and is returned uphill to the heart through veins. The uphill trip requires a good deal of work. Some of the work is done by contractions of smooth muscle in the vein walls, but adequate venous return requires movement of leg muscles to perform venous pumping. The contracting leg muscles squeeze vein walls inward and push blood against the vein valves. The one-way valves are constructed so that the pressure closes the lower valve and pushes blood through the upper valve.

Muscle activity in the chest, from breathing and from arm and head movement, also helps pump venous blood toward the heart and brain. Without leg movement, pressure from blood pooling in leg veins rises from 24mmHg (walking) to 90mmHg (standing still) in about 30 seconds. The increased pressure causes fluid leakage from veins into tissue spaces. As much as 15 to 20 percent of blood volume is lost in the first 15 minutes of standing still. The reduced venous return causes the heart to beat faster, trying to maintain adequate circulation.

Veins can be damaged by high pressure and blood pooling from prolonged inactivity while standing or sitting. The overstretched veins are unable to contract and the pooled venous blood can then be seen in a condition known as "varicose veins." Support hose, massage, and walking exercise can be helpful.

The relationship between blood pooling and clotting is understandable when we consider that blood contains clotting agents for wound-healing purposes. These agents (fibers) tend to form clots in slow moving or stationary blood. Clots also form around any rough, irregular surface (e.g., an injury or cholesterol deposit). The reader may get some ideas at this point of possible connections that may exist between inactivity, diet, and health. It is known already that leisurely walking, when done with regularity, can raise the level of "good" cholesterol (Duncan, Gordon, and Scott 1991).

Hypertension, or high blood pressure, is less frequent in people who engage in some form of exercise on a regular basis. Three 10-minute periods of walking spread throughout the day are as good as one 30-minute session (DeBusk et al. 1990).

Dietary factors for computer workers

There are relationships between heart disease, hypertension, diet, and activity that are important for sedentary workers such as computer users to know about. For example, a heart attack victim usually has a buildup of cholesterol "plaque" clogging the coronary arteries. Coronary arteries provide nutrients and oxygen to the heart muscles.

When plaque builds up, the danger of complete arterial blockage escalates, because plaque can break loose and block blood flow. Also, blood tends to clot around ridges of cholesterol.

Bypass surgery and angioplasty, in which the surgeon literally cleans out the artery, are surgical treatments for heart disease. Blood thinners such as aspirin are sometimes prescribed as a quick response to an episode or as a preventive measure. But diet, exercise, and stopping smoking can reduce your risk significantly. For example, smoking a pack of cigarettes a day *doubles* the risk of a coronary as compared to the risk of a nonsmoker. Smoking can increase the risk of a coronary more then twentyfold if the smoker also has high blood pressure and high cholesterol (Orleans and Slade 1993).

Plaque buildup in arteries creates hypertension, which causes the heart to pump faster. It can also overstretch arteries and cause tissue death (e.g., stroke) due to insufficient oxygen or nutrients. Reducing your sodium intake and alcohol consumption can, along with exercise and dietary discretion, play a significant role in controlling blood pressure.

The dietary measures for controlling heart disease and blood pressure are not hard to remember, because they affect the tendency to deposit the fatty substance cholesterol in arteries. Low-density lipoprotein (LDL) is the "bad" kind of cholesterol that can stick to your artery walls. High density lipoprotein (HDL) is the "good" kind of cholesterol that actually removes LDL from artery walls and takes it to the liver for incineration. You can keep your LDL level down by minimizing your consumption of saturated fats, commonly found in red meat, butter, cheese, whole milk, and tropical oils (palm, palm kernel, coconut). Saturated fat is solid at room temperature. Other kinds of fats are not LDL-promoting. Mono-unsaturated fats, such as olive, canola, and peanut, do not increase LDL (the "bad") or decrease HDL (the "good"). Polyunsaturated fats (corn, safflower, and sunflower) lower both kinds of cholesterol.[2] Read food labels and use foods with mono-unsaturated fat.

2 Summary of the "Second Report of the National Cholesterol Education Program Expert Panel on Detection, Evaluation, and Treatment of High Blood Cholesterol in Adults," *Journal of the American Medical Association*, Vol. 269, No. 3, June 16, 1993, pp. 3015–3023.

There is good evidence that certain vitamins can reduce LDL. The antioxidant vitamins E, C, and beta carotene appear to prevent LDL from sticking to artery walls. A recent study of 120,000 nurses indicated 40 percent less heart disease when they took 100 mg. of vitamin E every other day for a few years.[3] Vitamin E is found in unsaturated fats such as vegetable oil, margarine, nuts and whole grains, seafood, and green leafy vegetables. Vitamin C is found in berries, melons, citrus fruits, asparagus, broccoli, peppers, potatoes, and tomatoes. Beta carotene is found in dark green vegetables such as broccoli, and orange fruits and vegetables such as carrots, cantaloupe, and nectarines.

Dr. Dean Ornish conducted a study showing artery clearing in heart disease patients who quit smoking and followed a program that included low-fat meals, reduction of alcohol intake, increased activity, yoga, and meditation.[4] The yoga and meditation may be a good way to control the effects of workplace stress that increase the incidence of CTD. Another recommended source provides a program for reducing your risk of heart disease, cancer, and some other illnesses by reducing your fat intake to 10 percent, getting mild but regular exercise, and relaxing more (Kurzwel 1993). Stopping smoking is important because the smoke lowers good cholesterol, and harsh chemicals in the smoke damage arteries. Cholesterol tends to deposit at these damage sites.

(Important cautionary note: A low-fat diet is not for everyone. Small children and diabetics, for instance, should not restrict fat intake too much. Consult your doctor on all diet and health matters; the comments in this book reflect current research but are not intended as medical advice and should not supplant the care of your doctor.)

The remainder of this section on dietary factors will consist of several easy-to-follow rules for low LDL eating[5] and a bibliography of books on healthy-heart eating by well-known heart surgeons. These

3 *Harvard Heart Letter*, September 1993, pp. 4–5.

4 D. Ornish, "Can Lifestyle Changes Reverse Heart Disease?" *Lancet*, vol. 236, July 21, 1990, pp. 129–133.

5 Excerpted with permission from *The Heart Care Guide*, Hall-Foushee Productions, Inc., Suite 214B, 1313 5th St. SE, Minneapolis, MN 55414, 1994.

materials should provide more adequate coverage of a subject that is of particular importance to office workers and computer users who get little exercise in their work.

➤ Choose lean red meats, chicken, turkey (no skin), and fish. Serving no bigger than a deck of cards (3 oz.).

➤ Eat fruit and vegetables every day. However, avocados, olives, and coconut are not fat-free.

➤ Eat at least one of the following each meal: bread, cereal, rice, pasta, potatoes.

➤ Use less than half the amount of fat or oil you usually use; that is, less than half of margarine, salad dressing, mayonnaise, or cooking oil.

➤ Don't use saturated fats such as butter, cream, solid shortening, whole-milk products, cheese, coconut, and palm oil. Use polyunsaturated fats instead, such as corn oil, soybean oil, cottonseed oil, safflower oil, sunflower oil, and margarine made with these oils.

➤ Eat four or fewer egg yolks per week, including those in baked goods and prepared dishes.

➤ Use low-fat dairy products such as skim milk, low fat yogurt, low-fat cheese (e.g., mozzarella).

⇨ Activity & intestinal pumping

Food and waste are normally moved through the human digestive-intestinal system by a combination of intestinal contractions (peristalsis) and whole-body movement, such as walking. With adequate bulk fiber in the diet these mechanisms are normally adequate. Fiber is important for people of all ages, for peristaltic contractions need bulk to push against in moving material through the system. See how much easier it is to swallow (peristalsis) a small pill if it is embedded in a charge of food or liquid.

A. Kilbom (1987) cites studies indicating that people in sedentary occupations (e.g., bank officers, accountants, engineers) have at least

1.6 times more colon cancer than people in active jobs. The difference does not appear to be due to dietary differences. The most widely held explanation is that exercise facilitates bowel action, resulting in more rapid elimination of fecal material. The material contains carcinogenic and irritating substances including digestive bile acids. Prolonged sitting and inactivity lead to delayed and incomplete elimination, allowing the irritating substances extended contact with bowel membranes. This permits infectious bacterial processes to start. Other gastro-intestinal disorders, such as diverticulosis infection, can be avoided by exercise and adequate fiber.

The relation between exercise and bowel function is known to long-distance runners, whose strenuous exercise sometimes leads to diarrhea. A readable paperback on gastro-intestinal health (Perkins 1992) recommends walking every day, and if you have a sedentary job, to make a point of getting up every hour and walking to some far point of your building and up and down some stairs.

Colon cancer is second only to lung cancer in causing cancer death in the United States, with about 110,000 new cases and 51,000 deaths per year. A recent comprehensive review of medical and epidemiological research (Potter et al. 1993) solidly confirms the link between occupational inactivity and colon cancer, and also cites a firm relationship between leisure time activity and reduced risk. They affirm the importance of dietary fiber for reducing risk, but expand this category to include vegetables and plant food in general as important for reducing risk.

Fiber not only increases stool bulk and, along with exercise, reduces transit time, but binds and removes bile acids. Potter (et al. 1993) mentions that fiber may have the additional preventive effect of fermenting into certain fatty acids that directly prevent cancer growth.

The ingestion of a high dietary percentage of fat, meat, and animal protein is highly correlated with colon cancer. Fat and meat in particular stimulate bile production. There are other correlates of colon cancer; for example, genetics, excess weight, alcohol consumption, and exposure to pollutants such as asbestos, pesticides, and herbicides. One additional correlate may be of particular interest to computer buffs who munch while they compute. Eating frequently increases risk. This may be due to the fact that bile acids are secreted with every intake of food.

In the light of current medical and epidemiological knowledge, it is important for computer workers, who get little activity from their work, to generate activity during and after work, and to include plant foods as a significant factor in their diet. They should also minimize snacking frequency, especially of fat and animal protein.

Regarding antioxidant vitamins; a recent study of Iowa women, ages 55–69, showed a negative relationship between colon cancer and vitamin E intake.[6] A, C, beta-carotene, and selenium supplements did not show this relationship.

We can speculate on another reason why women computer workers in particular should get plenty of exercise. Such activity is even more strongly associated with reduced risk in women. Exercise stimulates the production of hormones, such as estradiol, progesterone, prolactin, lutenizing hormone, and follicle-stimulating hormone. These hormones may be involved in reducing risk for women. Here is the speculation. These hormones are also important for conception and for sustaining a pregnancy, and there has been a lot of publicity about a possible link between extensive computer use and miscarriage and conception failure (which may be very early miscarriage). The inactivity accompanying heavy computer use could be a factor in miscarriage.

⇨ Activity & the lymphatic pump

The skin and openings of our body are penetrated throughout the day by viruses, bacteria, fungi, parasites, and toxic substances. The immune system of the body provides "police" cells (lymphocytes) that patrol these areas. They identify the molecular structure of the intruder and then multiply in sufficient numbers to overcome and

6 R. Bostick, J. Potter, P. McKenzie, T. Sellers, L. Kushi, K. Steinmetz, and A. Folsom, "Reduced Risk of Colon Cancer with High Intake of Vitamin E: The Iowa Women's Health Study," *Journal of Cancer Research*, 53(18), 1993, pp. 4230–4237.

destroy them. Vaccination is a manmade method of stimulating our lymphocytes to identify and arm against a specific disease invader. Lymphocytes also work to destroy cancerous cells that have been created by mutation, or by abnormal activation of cell growth.

The lymphocytes are located strategically close to invasion sites. For example, lymphoid tissue in the stomach and intestinal tract is close to invaders entering the gut. Lymph tissues in the throat and pharynx (tonsils and adenoids) are close to invaders entering through the mouth and nose. Skin invaders are intercepted by lymphocytes in the lymph nodes. Lymphocytes in the spleen and bone marrow are well-situated to intercept invaders in the blood stream (Guyton 1992).

The invaders are taken up by lymphatic capillary-pump cell arrangements, as illustrated in Fig. 4-4. The large invader molecules can enter, but not exit, through the pores of the lymph capillary. When the capillary walls are distended they contract and, with the

Figure 4-4

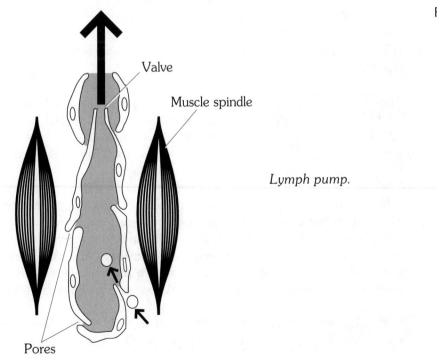

Valve

Muscle spindle

Lymph pump.

Pores

help of muscle contraction, push fluid upward in the system. Invader particles are destroyed as they pass through the lymph nodes.

Pressure on lymphatic vessels by contraction of muscles controlling limbs and breathing plays a significant role in moving fluid through the lymphatic system, increasing flow ten to thirtyfold. Thus, the lack of large muscle activity throughout the day can reduce resistance to disease.

Potter (et al. 1993) mentioned that activity is also important for maintaining immune-system vigor by stimulating the growth of antibody factors such as T cells, B cells, natural killer cells, and interleukin-1.

⇨ Activity & bone strength

An important general characteristic of people is their design for movement. This point is represented again in the fact that bone makes up over 40 percent of human body mass. Those bones and muscles are made for movement, and the bone is constantly being reshaped and reinforced to best support the owner's recent activity pattern.

That last sentence may seem a bit puzzling to those readers who tend to think of bone as an inactive, passive, or dead material, like concrete. Actually, bone is a live, active tissue that is constantly being destroyed and rebuilt to meet the owner's need for action and support.

It is another one of many interesting facts of physiology that there are cells, called osteoclasts, that are constantly at work removing bone from outer surfaces and from holes they dig inside the bone (Guyton 1992). Functionally they resemble that voracious character of early video games, Pac-Man® (with the big mouth), who chomped everything that didn't get out of the way fast enough (Fig. 4-5).

Cells with an appetite like Pac-Man®, osteoclasts work fast. They can eat (actually, dissolve with acid) out a tunnel up to 1 millimeter in

Figure 4-5

Pac-Man®, alluding to osteoclasts.

diameter and several millimeters long within three weeks. They are working on about four percent of the surface of adult bone at any given time. Normally this rapid loss of bone is balanced by the action of cells (osteoblasts) that deposit new bone. Osteoblasts tend to work at sites where bone strength is needed—at pressure sites and along stress lines created by movement. This is the way that bone is remodeled to improve support of the owner's movement pattern. Inactivity lends rather rapidly to progressive bone weakening (osteoporosis) and increases the likelihood of bone fracture and breakage. Movement involving compression of the long bones, as in walking, is the only kind of activity that prevents progressive bone loss and weakness (Kilbom 1987). The bone weakness appears in spinal bones as well as in other bones.

Body movement, seating, & the "ergonomically correct" chair

The great importance of body movement, including walking and posture variation during the work day, requires that we place additional emphasis on the dynamic chair back that is appearing now on some chair models. Some research needs to be done to see if any benefit issues from combining settable angles, or settable angle limits, with this design, but it is not too soon to make this an essential ergonomic specification for new seating.

The expression "ergonomic chair," or "ergonomically correct chair" is often used. This writer has yet to see a chair without a serious ergonomic deficiency. Some chairs have several desirable features; others have none or maybe just one. No one chair meets the criteria considered in Chapter 2. But chair design is still in the early stages of development, and improvements will come as long as the pressure for worker health continues.

The ANSI/HFS seating standard is also in the process of development. The first version (1988) has a lot of loopholes: hard arms are not ruled out, nothing was said about the importance of backward tilt, adjustable back support, settable or dynamic backs, the chair back does not have to support the upper body, and it does not have to fit the user. A chair that meets ANSI-HFS standards may have a few good features but it may also be a very bad chair, with hard arms, a rigid back, no lumbar cushion, and other deficiencies.

We hope that new versions of the standard will suggest that a variety of chairs that differ in pan height and size, arm height and style (no hard, slippery arms, please), back width, and back-support prominence will be made available for fit to individual workers. The standard should specifically recommend against requiring all workers to use the same model of chair. Health and safety features, such as padded arms and back tilt, should be no more optional than brakes or headlights on automobiles.

⇨ Chair selection

A variety of chair models and sizes should be collected together, reviewed for presence of ergonomic features and options, and then tried by workers before purchase. Some individuals will want and use models with many manual controls; others will want theirs to be as automatic as possible. Some chairs will fit no one; return these. Some individuals will fit none of the chairs; you widen the search for their benefit. Some individuals will be fussy and make sure they select the best chair for themselves; others will be willing to settle for anything you give them. Don't take advantage of the latter category. They may feel uncomfortable with this attention and self-concern, but you have a stake in their health. Make sure they try many models before choosing.

⇨ The importance of exercise during the work day

It is now commonly known that some vigorous form of exercise can make us healthier in many ways, by improving circulation, increasing muscle tone, and stimulating a more positive attitude. That is good news, but the main point of this chapter is that the predominance of sitting and inactivity in the office work environment has destructive effects on health, and that large muscle activity, such as walking for three or four five- to ten-minute periods per half day, are required to simply *maintain* one's current health condition. In addition, such exercise does reduce physiological and mental fatigue and stress, and increases energy and the capacity for work.

It is common for pamphlets and popular articles on office ergonomics to recommend simple exercises, either stretching or stretching and standing, that can be done sitting and/or standing without leaving the chair or the office work station. For example, you drop a pencil on the floor and pick it up, rotate your shoulders, and flex and point your feet and toes (Austin 1984). A recent short-term test of this proposal (Swanson and Sauter 1993) found that simple stretching exercises like these did not decrease reported discomfort in hand, wrist, arm, neck, or back, and did not improve mood, which grew more negative during the day.

However, there are reports that companies with stretching exercise programs do experience a reduction in medical and workers' compensation costs for some types of disorders that are caused by postural fixity and repetitive motion (Herbert 1992). It may be a matter of the specific stretching exercises and duration of program that determine effectiveness. Anyone who has ever driven a car for an hour or two straight before stopping at a rest area or gas station knows the relief that can be obtained from getting out of a posturally fixed position, stretching the back and shoulders, and walking about for as little as five minutes. The relief is from drowsiness and visual tension as well as muscle and skeletal discomfort. Such relief is usually adequate to refuel another hour of work.

Apply this experience to your own office work and that of your employees. Looking at a computer for hours is a lot like driving a car for hours, except that computer work requires repetitive strain on arms, wrists, and fingers, in addition to postural rigidity and visual strain. Also, car seats that allow you to lean back are easier on your spine than most office seating. A five-minute break from keyboarding every hour for stretching exercise will help some, but we can get

63

much more out of a break than that. A rest period spent sitting on a sofa in a lounge will do little except provide mental relief. Active walking, going up and down a flight or two of stairs in the process, will be a more productive way to spend break time.

Get rid of the lounge; there's already too much sitting in the average office. Deliver a message or two by hand rather than by e-mail. Use a rest room on another floor at least five minutes away. Encourage and reinforce your employees in doing the same. Fortuitous networking is another unappreciated benefit of face-to-face social exchanges between colleagues during the day.

Employee activities after work can help promote, or prevent, negative health outcomes of VDT activity during the work day. Unfortunately, a worker may be a couch potato (Democrat spelling) or potatoe (Republican spelling) at home (Actually, both are correct spellings!), or may spend much of his in-home time on a home computer. There is some evidence that workers with dominant interests in computers do a lot of computer game-playing and programming at home, and have little or no interest in exercise or sports (Shotton 1989). We can only hope that encouraging regular exercise at work will have some carryover into activities at home.

Unplanned networking among employees during the day has to be a major, generally unappreciated, productivity booster. Employees meet in the hallways and poke their noses into each other's cubicles. They meet in the mail room and over the coffee pot. Yet they talk about weather, newspaper and television reports, sports, their kids, and vacations. How can this be a productivity *booster*?

First of all, let us never forget that social approval and respect is the primary fuel that fires the engine of human productivity. It is communicated most effectively in personal, face-to-face exchange. People are in large part working for the approval and respect of others. If the work environment is to be a place where human industry, ingenuity, and loyalty are found in abundance, then it will be a place where people see and talk to each other every day. They follow a comment about the weather, or an expression of interest in the family, with an inquiry about how a certain project is progressing, or if there is a need for information or a contact. A kudo for a well-done job may be given. Invariably these days, information will be exchanged on how to solve software problems, or suggestions for more effective software programs.

Although frequent nose-poking into other workers' cubicles is not a productivity booster in and of itself, new projects, new solutions, cooperative working relationships, helpful information, useful contacts, encouragement to persist, advice on dealing with a person or situation—all these can emanate from interactions that occur primarily because they are social. Genuine good will and respect are often traded, sometimes by cues as subtle as a slight smile, a wrinkle of an eye, or a second look. It's very difficult to do this on e-mail, but e-mail does have its own uses.

You can facilitate constructive networking by setting aside an area where tools and equipment like the copy machine, printer, fax, and coffee pot will bring people together. If you are a manager or supervisor, join in the hallway or coffee room conversations. Joining in could save you from believing a really dumb idea—for example, that the employees are just "goofing off." Joining in can also be an excellent, informal way to follow progress on projects and provide encouragement. It can also discourage the few who might be inclined to goof off.

We were surprised to learn that exercise periods during the day were recommended as productivity boosters in management texts near the turn of the century. For example, *Scientific Office Management*, by W. H. Leffingwell (1917), includes accounts of how companies like Willys-Overland, Curtis Publishing, Montgomery Ward, Remington Typewriter, The Chicago Ferrotype Company, and various telephone companies had found that rest and exercise periods during the day boosted productivity. The book includes pictures of employees doing exercises at their desks, similar to what we have seen in Japanese offices. Leffingwell was a proponent of the efficiency and productivity teachings of Frederick W. Taylor. He lamented the fact that too few managers ". . . are wise enough freely to grant rest periods to employees." His discussion of the potential problems in requiring employees to take rest/exercise breaks is interesting.

In the Chicago Ferrotype Company the employees were urged to go outside and play during recess. At first there were some who preferred to sit and relax at their desks, but the management felt that a little physical exercise would be better and therefore made it a rule that employees must take the recess and made it very evident that it preferred them to take a walk outside. One of the leading business men of Detroit, to whom this was told, said that this was neither more nor less than slavery. "The company has no right to compel an employee to go outside, or to rest, even on the grounds that it is for his personal interest to do so," said he. That may be so, but if this attitude is taken, neither has the company a right to compel its employees to come to work at a certain hour, nor to work a certain number of hours, nor to accept a certain wage. As a matter of fact the compulsion is of a subtle nature, since the employee is apparently free to refuse to work at all under any conditions, but if a company is to be criticized for compelling its employees to take recreation, how much more should it be criticized for compelling them to work? (pp. 44–45)

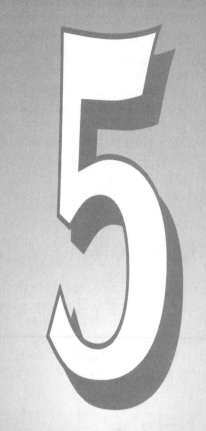

CTDs of the upper extremities & workstation accommodations

W E presented some material on cumulative trauma disorders (CTDs) in Chapter 3, which dealt primarily with seating. That material emphasized how a slumped or fixated seating posture can lead to developing CTDs in the upper body as well as the lower spine area. This chapter will describe some of the CTDs in more detail and suggest some workstation adjustments to help reduce the CTD-causing potential of a computer workstation. Carpal tunnel syndrome will be described first because it is the most publicized CTD, although it is not the most frequently occurring one.

⇨ Keyboard location

Given the importance of varied seating posture, from 120 degrees (leaning back) to 90 degrees (upright), it is important to put the keyboard on a movable and tiltable tray or surface that can be adjusted to a new location when the worker changes position. It is important that the worker use the keyboard in a wrist-neutral posture without lifting up with shoulders and arms, and without reaching for it.

⇨ Keyboard height

First of all, the keyboard has to be high enough to permit the legs to fit underneath. Figure 5-1 shows an alternative solution to the problem of getting close to the keyboard and mouse without leaning forward—side-saddle keyboarding. But she won't hold out long in that position. This is a bad workstation design.

It is important that the keyboard be adjustable in height, as well as location and tilt, so that it can be used in an arm- and wrist-neutral position. Repetitive, prolonged keyboarding, over weeks or months, can be a factor leading to carpal tunnel syndrome or another cumulative trauma disorder. Surveys and studies consistently show CTDs to be a function of keyboarding frequency and duration. CTD is more likely to occur when the worker's wrists are bent and/or flexed to the task. Dr. David Rempel of the University of California, San Francisco, presented data at the Marconi Keyboard Research

Figure 5-1

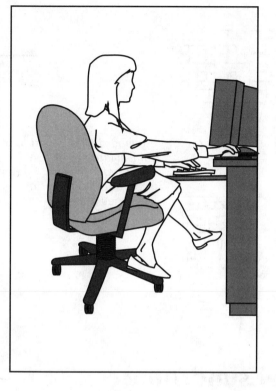

Side-saddle keyboarder.

Conference[1] showing that typing with wrists extended up actually increased carpal tunnel pressure.

Carolyn Sommerich and Dr. William Mappas of Ohio State University presented work at the same conference showing that typing with a split keyboard (no ulnar deviation) reduced CTP. Figure 5-2 shows how separating keys for left and right hands allows keying from a less deviated wrist position. The separated keys are on a kinesis keyboard.[2]

ANSI/HFS 100 (1988) agrees with the importance of maintaining a comfortable arm angle and, in general, an adjustability range of 23 to 28 inches (p. 47).

1 Marconi Keyboard Research Conference, Marshall, CA, February 18-19, 1994, reported in *VDT News*, May/June 1994, p. 4.

2 Kinesis Corp., 915 118th Ave. SE, Bellevue, WA 98005-3855, 206-455-9220.

Figure 5-2

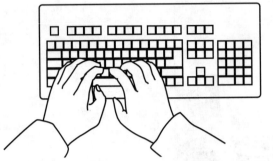

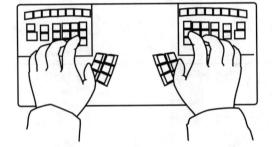

Keyboard wrist positions.
(a) Deviated wrists on
standard keyboard. (b) Key
separation eliminating
wrist deviation. Kinesis

⇨ Carpal tunnel syndrome

Bent-wrist keyboarding can lead to carpal tunnel syndrome because the median nerve passes through a tunnel that has wrist (carpal) bones on three sides and a ligament on the palm side. The tunnel is small, with the approximate diameter of the tip of your little finger. The median nerve is crowded into the tunnel with flexor tendons that control thumb and finger movement, and many blood vessels and ligaments.

The muscles that move your fingers and your wrist are located in your forearms. The finger bones are connected to these muscles by tendons passing through the carpal tunnel. Rapid, frequent, stereotyped finger and thumb movements can cause chafing, irritation, and inflammation of these tendons, especially when a bent or flexed wrist causes them to move against each other and the carpal bones.

Figure 5-3 shows the median nerve passing through the tunnel and innervating the thumb, pointer, and middle fingers, and inside of the ring finger. Figure 5-4 shows tendons rubbing against bones of the forearm and flexed wrist.

The tendons are surrounded by synovial sheaths, which exude a lubricating agent called synovial fluid. The fluid protects tendons from chafing and irritation in the course of normal, nonintensive finger, thumb, and wrist movements. Keystroking at high rates, for hours at a time, over months, exceeds the lubricating capabilities of tendon sheaths. They were simply not designed for that. Chafed, irritated tendons become inflamed and swollen, which, along with excess synovial fluid, creates a buildup of pressure within the narrow carpal tunnel. The building pressure will eventually press hard enough on the median nerve to cause nerve compression, which you know from hitting your "funny bone" (ulnar nerve) near your elbow.

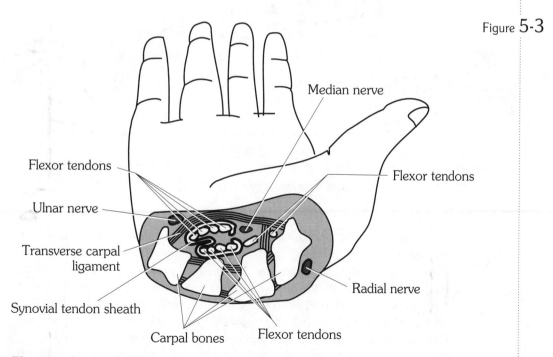

Figure 5-3

The carpal tunnel. Wrist section showing bones, ligaments, tendons, and nerves.

Figure 5-4

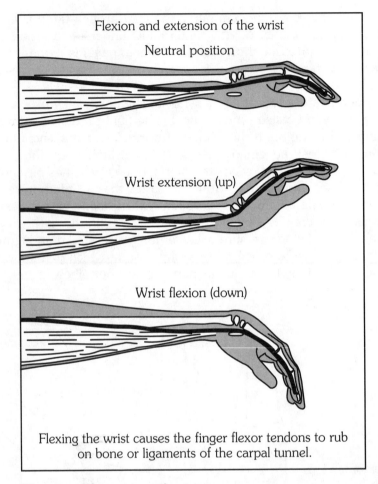

Flexion and extension of the wrist

Neutral position

Wrist extension (up)

Wrist flexion (down)

Flexing the wrist causes the finger flexor tendons to rub on bone or ligaments of the carpal tunnel.

Flexing and extension of wrist.

The sudden nerve compression of hitting your ulnar nerve caused strong symptoms: sharp tingling, pain, numbness, weakness, and disability. You can imagine how unpleasant and disabling it would be to have those same symptoms around the clock when abused tendons have created persisting high pressure in the carpal tunnel. Often the pain is strongest at night, when swelling is greatest. Abused tendons, muscles, and nerves in other parts of the keyboarding-involved anatomy also produce pains of inflammation and nerve compression at other sites, some of which are described at the end of this section.

The important point here is that upper-extremity CTDs are not separate "diseases" at all. They are simply vulnerable points in a tightly packed, intertwined network of blood vessels, bones, tendons, nerves, and muscles, where these elements sometimes rub against hard corners of bone, or have been squeezed between expanding, contracting, twisting knots of muscle. Parts of the network passing through gauntlets of scissoring and sawing tendons might have stretched to the point of fraying, or are buffeted and compressed by external objects where they come close to the skin.

It is remarkable how these sinewy appendages—our arms and hands—perform, from microsurgery to Svjatoslav Richter's playing of Beethoven's *Emperor* Concerto, or Larry Bird's sinking of 20 three-pointers in a row. It is not surprising that some problems develop at points of suspension and intersection, when the elements are forced to operate repetitively for hours on end, over months and years, from contorted and fixated postures. They were designed more for complex work than for machine-gun repetition.

Several physical conditions predispose a given individual to develop carpal tunnel syndrome from keyboarding, among them arthritis, diabetes, gout, hypothyroidism, pregnancy, female gender, birth control pills, menopause, wrist size, strongly muscled thick wrists, obesity, Lyme disease, and some medications used in treating depression.

Several studies have linked overweight (obesity) to slowed conductivity of the median nerve (Allen 1993). Among the mechanisms for this relationship is the greater body width of obese workers, which leads to greater ulnar wrist deviation in keyboard use.

(For your own information, the formula for calculating obesity was a body mass index (BMI), derived by dividing body weight in kg by the square of height in meters (BMI=kg/m2). Thus a BMI of 21 or less was considered "slender"; 21.1 to 24.9 equaled "medium"; 25 to 30 equaled "overweight"; and over 30 equaled "obese.")

If keyboard activity is reduced or eliminated when the symptoms first appear the symptoms will gradually go away. Continuing to keyboard at high rates, despite the pain, will cause pressure to build up high enough to squash, and permanently damage, the median nerve. Thus it is important to stop or significantly modify the abusive keyboard activity as soon as the first symptoms appear. Do not continue until pain and disability force you to stop.

If you supervise keyboard workers, you or a trained delegate must get to know them, gain their trust, and stay tuned-in to their physical condition. You must create a trusting environment that encourages the reporting of pains and does not punish individuals who develop them. It makes good business sense to do this, for treating a fully developed disorder such as carpal tunnel is very expensive, and full recovery of function is not likely. Surgery for one wrist generally costs $5,000 to $10,000, but the total direct and indirect costs of the injury may range between $10,000 and $60,000. The surgery, which may involve severing the carpal ligament in order to release pressure, leaves the hand in a weakened condition.

Creating trust and a caring environment is not the only way to generate a readiness to complain. Studies consistently show that workers who distrust their management and think their supervisors don't care about their health are more likely to complain. They are also more likely to seek compensation. There are additional problems with the uncaring approach: the costs will probably be higher than with a caring approach, for workers will seek compensation as a way out from under the supervisor rather than trying to work with the company to improve conditions before compensation is necessary. Also, with uncaring supervision there will be some individuals who view not complaining and working with pain as loyalty to the company. They will have the most serious injuries.

⇨ Vitamins

There are some encouraging indications that vitamins may help treat cumulative trauma such as carpal tunnel syndrome. A ten-year research project by Karl Folkers, Director of the Institute for Biomedical Research at the University of Texas (Folkers 1986), indicated that individuals with CTD, regardless of age or gender, have a marked deficiency in vitamin B6 (pyridoxine). They may or may not be eating well and getting normal amounts of B6 daily; but for reasons of individual biochemistry they are deficient in the enzymes that require B6 for synthesis. Large doses of B6, over two to three months, have been effective. The combination of B6 with B2 (riboflavin) has been most effective. B2 is required to convert oral B6 into an effective form. Folkers reported on some patients with carpal tunnel syndrome who had surgery on one hand, then developed the disorder in the other hand. Both hands showed a positive response to B6. Folkers recommended taking the B6 and B2 supplements as a preventive.

Some physicians are also reporting success with B6. For example, Dr. Morton Kasdan of Louisville, Kentucky, is using B6, along with modification of activity and wrist splints worn at night, to treat most of his patients. However, he cautions that too much B6 can be dangerous (Assembly 1988). Dr. Peter Nathan also reports a role for vitamin B6 in reducing symptoms of carpal tunnel syndrome.[3]

Vitamins C and E in large doses, under medical supervision, have been reported as helpful in treating carpal tunnel syndrome and synovial sheath irritation, in cases that have been detected early, with sensory disturbance only, before muscle weakness or atrophy (Marsh and McClennan 1983). Vitamin C is an anti-inflammatory agent, and vitamin E helps circulation and prevents scarring.

Thus, early detection of CTD symptoms, plus conservative treatment consisting of modification of the abusive activity and insistence on workers' taking active work breaks every hour, may allow effective treatment with the outlay of only a few dollars for vitamins instead of expensive surgery and the likelihood of some disability. It seems worth a try, although surgically oriented physicians may be reluctant to recommend it.

3 P. A. Nathan, "Carpal Tunnel Syndrome: Is it Caused by work?" 1994 Symposium, *Cumulative Trauma of the Upper Extremity*, American Association for Hand Surgery, Bloomington, MN.

Poor keyboard technique

Improving keyboarding technique can also help treat and prevent CTD. Pascarelli and Kella (1993) used videotape to study the keyboard technique of fifty-three CTD sufferers. Most were women ranging in age from 23 to 63 years; half as many were men, ranging in age from 25 to 54 years. Thirty-four were writers, journalists, or editors. The rest were typists, word processors, programmers or systems analysts, a graphic artist, a typesetter, and a telemarketer.

The most common pains in this group were of the forearm, elbow, wrist, and thumb. A surprising 72 percent had some hypermobile (back-bending) joints in some or all of their fingers, including their thumbs. Forty-three percent used dorsiflexed (flexed upward) wrists while keying; 38 percent used ulnar deviation (bent outward) wrists. Obesity increased the ulnar deviation. For 83 percent, one or both thumbs were held in an extended position during keying, whether they were used to hit the space bar or not. This appeared to be a way to keep the thumb out of the way and ready for action during keying, but this rigidity made flexing the other fingers harder.

Sixty-four percent presented a hyperextended fixed fifth finger (the little finger) in both hands, even though it was not used to strike any keys. When used for keying it was used to strike offset function keys.

Joint hypermobility increases keying difficulty; thus these individuals tended to key with stiffened fingers. Women with long fingernails typed this way too, because they did not strike the keys with their fingertips. The consequence of hypermobile digits, whether stiffened or not, was extra wrist action during keying. Long fingernails also led to extra wrist flexion.

Hypermobile-jointed persons were taught to strike keys from a slightly flexed, not stiffened, position, to prevent joint collapse when striking a key. Twenty-six percent hit the keys with excessive force, which could be detected by the loud clacking noises their keyboards made when the keys were struck.

These individuals can be trained to use less force, of course, but there are also new keyboards out that require less force to operate and their keys don't bottom-out with as much impact. For example, clients trying out the new keytronics keyboards report that they are, as advertised, easier to key.[4]

There were some hunt-and-peck typists in the Pascarelli study, along with the majority of more-or-less touch typists. The hunters (three men) used their two strongest fingers, the index and middle fingers. Videotapes showed them using a lot of wrist flexion, up and down, when keying, as well as a lot of left and right sideways wrist deviation when traveling to keys. They were slow, and so were less seriously injured than the others.

The worst-case keying scenario for the touch-typers had them reaching for keys by lifting their wrists up, flexing their wrists down and striking the keys with their wrists in a rigid bent-sideways position, with a hyperextended thumb and middle finger. They were also dealing with the problems that attend hypermobile finger joints. For example, they flexed their wrists down while striking keys, and after striking keys they flexed their wrists upward again.

Pascarelli and Kella also discussed the biomechanical demands of using a mouse. They mentioned the double-click requirement, as well as the tendency to pinch the mouse between the index finger and thumb. They also mentioned the injury potential of placing the mouse too high or too low.

We've found that heavy mouse use is often associated with wrist pain. Trackballs also seem to create problems. Mouse usability could be improved by increasing the gain, so that a full screen transit could be achieved by about one inch of mouse transit.

Many alternative cursor control devices are available, including un-mouses and spaceballs. But two others seem to have promise. The first, available through Felix Contact Altra in Wyoming, uses finger

4 Keytronic, P. O. Box 14687, Spokane, WA 99214-0687.

control to achieve full screen transit with about 1½ inches at control transit.[5]

A promising new control employs force-sensitive-resistor (FSR) technology. The user need only apply a light pressure in the direction of cursor movement desired. No wrist deviation is required. One IBM-compatible version of this device is made by Interlink Company and is called Versapoint.[6] It uses a small, dished-out button that is pressed with one finger. Cursor control is fast, smooth, and precise. This initial finger-based control should evolve into a more comfortable device in the near future. Versapoint was difficult to install on the computer, but FSR may be the technology of the future for cursor control, and it should help reduce wrist pain.

Pascarelli and Kella barely scratch the surface on the study of individual technique in keyboard work. Some workers habitually keyboard with neck, shoulder, or arm muscles in a persisting state of isometric contraction, which has been associated with tendonitis and muscle pain in these areas (Sommerich, McGlothlin, and Marras 1993). The worker could be taught to relax these muscles while keyboarding, and to take many small "micro" breaks during intensive keying.

One last word about carpal tunnel syndrome. This particular condition is difficult to diagnose. A symptom of wrist pain is not diagnostic. People have been known to complain of carpal tunnel syndrome after using a hand tool for a few hours. If it were carpal tunnel, it would not be caused by a few hours of tool use. Medical knowledge and experience are required to diagnose the various CTDs. Pain in wrists and forearms can be symptomatic of tendonitis (inflamed tendons), tenosynovitis (swollen tendon sheaths), or other conditions. For example, it is not uncommon for keyboard workers to develop tendonitis from resting wrists on the sharp edge of a desk top while keyboarding. Carpal tunnel syndrome can even occur without the element of repetitive motion.

5 Felix Contact Altra, 1200 Skyline Drive, Laramie, WY 82070, 307-745-7538.

6 Interlink Electronics, 546 Flynn Road, Camarillo, CA 93012.

The Pinsky book (1993) provides a readable account of some questions you can ask and simple tests you can conduct in order to get some idea of the location of your arm, wrist, or hand pain prior to seeing a physician. Don't diagnose yourself, however; CTD diagnosis is a very complicated affair and requires a specialist, and a very patient specialist at that. For more detail on carpal tunnel syndrome and other CTDs associated with keyboarding, the book by Pascarelli and Quilter (1994) is recommended as most authoritative.

Wrist braces and splints that constrict wrist movement are sometimes worn by people doing a lot of wrist work. Braces and splints are helpful in the healing process after surgery, but should not be worn at the first tinge of pain, or as a means of preventing carpal tunnel syndrome. Keyboarding with a splint will force the use of arms and shoulders in awkward positions.

One more point about wrist splints. They are not always properly fitted. Often the patient just gets a package of splints and puts them on. A poorly fitted splint may be abandoned because it hurts; if worn it can lead to contorted arm and shoulder movements. Pascarelli and Quilter recommend against using splints while working. In fact, OSHA law forbids the use of splints during work (OSHA document 3123).

⇨ Wrist pads

Foam pads are often recommended for supporting wrists (the heel of the hand, to be more precise) while keyboarding or using a mouse. They are helpful if they prevent wrists from contacting sharp desk or table edges and if they raise wrists level with the surface of the keyboard, so that keying can be done with straight wrists. Flat pads put less pressure on wrists than curved ones.

Keyboard workers seem to always have the legs up on the back of their keyboard, which causes the keyboard to slope down toward the worker. This sloped keyboard attitude is not recommended, for it requires wrist bent upwards (i.e. wrist "extension") to reach the back keys as illustrated in Fig. 5-5. If the keyboard is used in a more level

Figure 5-5

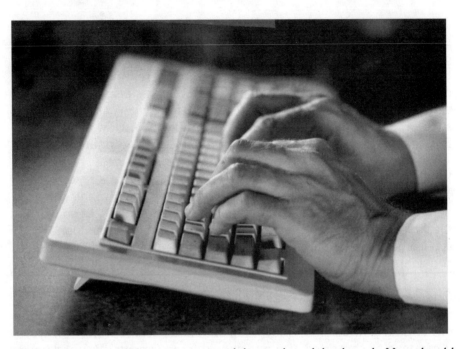

The poor wrist position necessitated by a sloped keyboard. You should flatten the keyboard.

attitude, then a foam wrist rest can help create a neutral, unflexed wrist position. How can we straighten out the poor wrist position in Fig. 5-5? Flatten out the keyboard and put a flat foam pad under the heels of the hands.

ANSI/HFS 100 (1988) recommends that keyboard slope be minimized and kept between 0 percent and 15 percent at most, p. 37.

If your keyboard activity requires keying in a given sequence of characters or words many times during the day, then a macro program can save you a lot of keystrokes. These programs can remember a variety of keyboard activities, such as drawing graphics, menu choices, and mouse movements in addition to text. The program remembers the sequence and runs it off automatically when you hit a function key. Hit F10, for example, to print your name, address, and directions to your house or place of business. Programs for keyboard remapping will also let you do the same thing.

Video display unit location & support surface adjustability

If the keyboard worker is going to vary seating posture, then the monitor-viewing angle will have to be easily adjustable for comfortable viewing from the different postures. Tilting monitor mounts are readily obtained from any computer supply store.

Generally, video units should not be mounted on top of the computer/drive unit if both are placed on a desk. This writer has relieved many sore, kinked necks by simply lowering the video unit to the desk so that the operator does not look up at the screen (See Fig. 5-6.)

Operators who wear bifocals will need their monitors lowered, because they have to crane their necks back to look straight ahead.

Figure 5-6

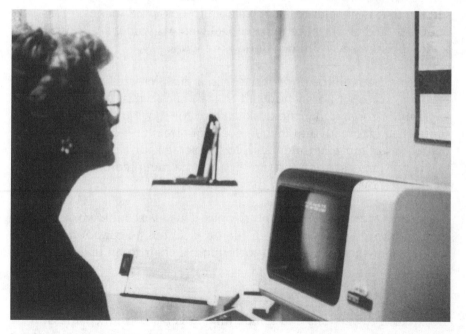

Looking at the display through bifocals.

You can recommend that they get special glasses with lenses ground for a specific focal length for monitor viewing, but not all will take the initiative to do it.

One negative feature of most glasses is that they are usually ground for a focal length farther away than the monitor. Thus, moving close enough to read the characters takes the characters out-of-focus.

People tend to have a shorter focal length when looking down at objects than when looking straight ahead (Kroemer, Kroemer, and Kroemer-Elbert 1994). Thus, it may be more comfortable looking down at a small monitor than looking ahead at it, or looking at a monitor while leaning back than while sitting upright. Chapter 10 contains more material on vision and glasses.

One recommendation is that the height as well as the tilt of monitors should be adjustable. The user who must use bifocals may want to lower the monitor base below the common desk height of 28 to 29 inches. There are suppliers who can provide a monitor-support surface that is tiltable and is adjustable to below 28 inches.[7] This option should be very useful to bifocal wearers who want to vary their seated posture several times during the work day.

Mounting the monitor on a desk, or in a desk, creates viewing problems for operators who want to lean back while keying. If there is plenty of room under the desk surface for moving thighs and arm supports underneath and maybe even for stretching of legs, then the operator can move close enough to the screen for clear viewing. If this is not the case then the monitor can be mounted on an arm that will allow moving it closer to the worker.

Desks are often too low for tall people. This causes the worker to slump forward when working at the desk. Often he cannot get his thighs under the table without lowering his chair to an uncomfortable level.

Adjustable tables are available from any furniture supply store. There are motorized versions and handcranking versions that cost less. If

7 Nova Office Furniture Inc., 421 West Industrial Avenue, Effingham, IL 62401.

you don't like the idea of throwing away a table or desk in good condition, and want to save a few dollars, try converting it to a height-adjustable model with a conversion kit.[8]

ANSI/HFS 100 (1988) recommends an under-desk leg clearance of 26.2 inches for nonadjustable surfaces. It recommends a range of 20.2 to 26.2 inches for adjustable surfaces, pp. 44–45.

Twenty-six inches of under-desk height will produce a desk that is too high for short people. The only practical solution is an adjustable surface, or a surface that can be mounted at a chosen height on a system panel. There must be adequate space under the surface for stretching out legs. Removing pencil drawers from desks helps solve the problem for some workers.

⇨ Automating (re-engineering) computer work

There is no doubt that we live in the computer age. Many kinds of work are done so much faster now. Computers enable workers in some fields to do much more than before. Engineers, graphic designers, and architects can design in three dimensions. Mathematical and statistical solutions have never been as fast and accurate as they are now on computers. E-mail is a breeze, and word processing programs have taken a lot of the frustration out of writing, though some with one foot still stuck in old world ways try to cc people with e-mail. True, prolonged keyboarding can tax and injure, and reasonable guidelines for this are wanting, but many of the benefits of the computer age do not require keyboard work at all. For example, using ATMs and cash cards has made visits to the bank a lot easier and less embarrassing. Credit cards make it wonderfully easy to incur debt.

Calling in a catalog order is much faster now that your profile and credit history, and who knows what else, are on a database. When

---

8 The Movatec Retrofit Height Adjustment System by Suspa, Inc., 3970 Roger Chaffee Drive SE, Grand Rapids, MI 49548-3497.

the clerk has just three items of information, your telephone number, catalog number, and credit card number, your name and mailing address appear on the screen. With just a few more keystrokes the clerk can flash the information to the stockroom at the speed of light, and your order will be mailed out the same day, unless the company uses a just-in-time inventory-delivery system, which often means that you go on back order.

How much easier this is than in the old days when orders were put on paper, with copies routed by hand, and usually got screwed up somewhere by someone who couldn't print clearly, or who mistook a "b" for an "h," or who couldn't tell you at the time you ordered that they no longer carried that model or color. How much more convenient now to have your credit card rejected right in front of other shoppers than to bounce a check in private. A lot less paperwork for everyone concerned, and you don't have to pay a penalty. These are familiar examples of work that has been re-engineered, using computers to reduce the amount of manual handwork required to input and process transactions. Reduced manual data entry, whether hand printing or keyboarding, means greater speed and accuracy. Automatic data storage on computer media, such as optical discs, means greater speed and accuracy of filing and accessing records. Computer memory also takes up a lot less space than the filing cabinets once used to store paper records.

Re-engineering that reduces the amount of manual keyboard work in data entry or processing can reduce the frequency of CTD in computer-intensive work, as well as increase speed and accuracy. Scanning machines can substitute for manual data entry in many applications, and can handle a good portion of it in others. Data are input on a structured order form. A scanner reads printed characters and numbers in certain fields of the form; a mark sensor looks for marks, such as check marks or filled-in circles, in other parts of the form. Thus, an order that indicates part number, part description, quantity, price, delivery date, style, and color can be taken without any human keyboard activity at all. Exceptions to the standard order procedure are routed to an operator who can handle it. There are scanners that scan both sides of a form and can identify colors. Scanners are sometimes tailored for certain kinds of documents, such as checks (both sides), engineering drawings, and legal documents.

Scanners can input graphic drawings. Television cameras can act as scanners for three-dimensional objects. The video image is digitized and put in computer memory along with text and two-dimensional drawings.

Your fax machine can function as a scanner.[9] A faxed request for certain kinds of information can automatically trigger sending the information by fax, without any human intervention.

Microfilm records can be run through a video scanner, digitized, and stored on an optical disc for fast computer access. Optical character recognition (OCR) scanners are used to greatly reduce the keyboard work required for identifying and routing forms in forms-intensive businesses such as law firms, health care, banking, transportation, and manufacturing. Scanners can increase processing efficiency more than 60 percent in such applications. Bar code scanners can also be used for indexing and routing forms in these industries. Scanners and PC-based workstations can reduce the manual workload in any computer-intensive application. The equipment can be paid for by savings in workers' compensation costs, if this is an issue. Here are a couple of illustrations.

A health care insurance provider processed more than 60,000 medical forms for payment. A claim form was date stamped after receipt of the forms and was sent to data entry. There, an average of 750 keystrokes were required to enter the information into the database. The proper forms were filed nearby for reference. After re-engineering this job, the information from each form was scanned onto an optical disk and basic information, identified by OCR, was stored in a data file. Data input staff reviewed any records that had been flagged for exceptions, legibility, or missing information. The workload on data entry operators was reduced by 60 percent or more and was made more interesting. The space used for paper file cabinets was released for other uses.[10]

A California Tax Board uses OCR and character-recognition scanning to enter data from paper tax forms into its main computer. Operators

9 A fax applications company: Harvest Software, 320 Soquel Way, Sunnyvale, CA 94086, 408-245-2600, Fax 408-245-2030.

10 Application by Image Network Technology, 9661 Telstar Ave., Unita El Monte, CA 91731, 818-454-1617.

deal with records flagged for exceptions. Projections for 1994 estimated the processing of three million forms using this system.[11]

Not all keyboard-intensive data entry work is simple transfer of information from paper to computer memory. Court reporting, for example, requires a great deal of special training and equipment. Because of the high frequency and costs of CTD in court reporters, many county and municipal court systems are converting to audio recording of courtroom proceedings. Special tape recorders record from as many as eight different microphones, and put each microphone on a separate channel. They can record for as long as six hours without a tape change. Later, the court reporter types the proceedings from the taped material. Before audio recording, the reporter hand-typed court proceedings in real time using a special chord typewriter, and then retyped the material later to produce the court record.[12]

Oddly, reporters who do audio recording in court get paid less than do manual recorders. This is odd because such a policy provides an incentive for employees to continue using manual keyboards wherever possible, thus engaging continued hazards that will lead to personal injury and increase workers' compensation costs to the employer. A more reasonable policy would be to increase, or at least not reduce, pay to recorders who use audio recording in court and take employer savings and equipment costs out of reduced compensation costs and insurance premiums.

Speech recognition is now a usable data-input technology. The worker simply talks into a microphone and the computer obeys commands and prints the text in the proper field. Vocal cord fatigue will define limits of productivity with this approach. The following letter was dictated into a computer for me:

11 Application by Southern Computer Systems, Inc., P. O. Box 1888, Birmingham, AL 35201-1888, 205-251-2985.

12 Application by Precision Business Systems, Inc., 9201 E. Bloomington Freeway, Bloomington, MN 55420, 612-884-9011.

Speech Recognition Technologies, A Division of BMS
10500 Wayzata Boulevard, Minneapolis, MN 55305-1511
Tel (612) 544-6977 Fax (612) 593-9635

November 17, 1993

Richard L. Patten, Ph.D.

Dear Richard,

As we discussed, I am enclosing the following literature:

  A brochure describing DragonDictate-30K v2.0
  A brochure describing PowerSecretary.

DragonDictate-30K was originally announced in March, 1991. It is
the standard for large vocabulary, free-text speech recognition
systems. As I may have mentioned, most of today's large vocabulary
systems use Dragon Systems technology.

While DragonDictate is designed to operate on IBM or compatible
systems under DOS, PowerSecretary is a portation of DragonDictate
to the Macintosh platform.

Speech Recognition Technologies represents both of these systems in
Minnesota and surrounding areas.

Thank you for your advice. I know there are many employees who
need the capabilities offered by these systems.

Please let me know how I may be of further service.

Cordially,

Van B. Thompson
General Manager

PS: This letter was created in a few seconds with speech recognition.

Cumulative trauma disorders of the upper extremities

Cumulative trauma disorders (also called repetitive strain injuries) can
involve stress and damage to tendons, tendon sheaths, ligaments,
muscles, nerves, and blood vessels in the neck, arm, hand, and
fingers. Tendon problems are most common.

Tendons connect muscle to bone; they have little elasticity, so excessive pressure, or prolonged constant pressure, will cause small tears which lead to inflammation and pain. Repeated rubbing against bone or other tissue can also lead to tendon inflammation (tendonitis).

Tendons are protected and suspended by sheaths where they must turn a corner. For example, the small extensor tendons that lift the fingers and wrist pass through sheaths. Repeated lifting up of fingers and wrist, or rigidly holding them up, can lead to tears in the tendon and thus to tendonitis (see extensor tendonitis, no. 3 in Fig. 5-7).

DeQuervain's disease (no. 9) is a name for painful tendonitis that affects the thumb-extensor tendon where it passes through a sheath as it curves from the wrist to the thumb. The tendon and sheath irritation that result from frequently hitting the space bar hard with the thumb is one of several bad keying habits that can lead to this painful disorder. The sheath, damaged from excessive friction, tends to swell and produces excess synovial fluid which collects and presses on the extensor tendon, making tendon passage difficult and painful. Such a condition of tendon sheaths is called tenosynovitis. A person with DeQ's disease feels pain when the thumb is lifted or the hand is twisted.

Intersection syndrome (no. 8) refers to tenosynovitis at a place on the dorsal (top) forearm where wrist-extensor tendons and thumb-extensor tendons cross over each other. Repetitive work with wrist and thumb extended causes the crossing tendons and sheaths to rub against each other, which leads to swelling, fluid build-up, and pain.

Extensor tendonitis (no. 3) can result if the hand is held up, extended, for long periods of time, or is repeatedly lowered and lifted. Tendon damage and/or tenosynovitis can produce pain in the hand near the wrist. This is a common movement and a common affliction, for musicians as well as keyboard workers.

Medial epicondylitis (no. 6) is known around the links as "golfer's elbow." The muscles that flex the wrist (down) and pronate the forearm and hand (turning the palm down) attach with a short tendon to the medical epicondyl (the inside elbow bone). Repeated forceful forearm and hand pronation, or wrist flexion, can lead to tendonitis

Figure 5-7

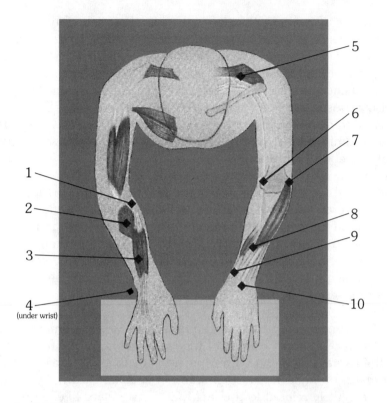

1. Cubital tunnel syndrome
2. Radial tunnel syndrome
3. Extensor Tendonitis
4. Carpal tunnel syndrome
5. Postural thoracic outlet syndrome

6. Medial epicondylitis
7. Lateral epicondylitis
8. Intersection syndrome
9. DeQuervain's disease
10. Distal P.I.N. syndrome

Locations of various muscle & nerve afflictions attributed to improper workstation use.

at the epicondyle. It can also lead to a bad hook. Mouse users tend to develop epicondylitis.

Lateral epicondylitis (no. 7) occurs where the muscles that extend the wrist (up) and supinate the forearm and the hand (turn the palm up) connect with a short tendon to the lateral (outside) epicondyle. Known as "tennis elbow," tendon tearing at the lateral epicondyle is common also in baseball pitchers and screwdriver users, and can be associated with certain keyboard habits.

Major nerves of the arm pass through several tunnels of bone, ligament, muscle, tendons, and other tissues as they wend their way down the arm to the hand. They also pass around moving edges of bone at the elbow. Swelling of surrounding tissue can compress nerves passing through the tunnels. Nerves passing around the elbow are also exposed to compression from external pressure. The nerve-compression disorders are often called "tunnel syndromes." We have already examined how the median nerve can be compressed at the carpal tunnel of the wrist.

Radial tunnel syndrome occurs when radial nerve compression at or near the lateral epicondyle comes from bone contact or muscle contraction. Pain occurs at the lateral epicondyle when the middle finger is extended. This syndrome can be confused with tennis elbow, but it must be treated before the nerve is damaged. Thus, you should not try to diagnose your own disorders. You could confuse these two and permit serious nerve damage. See a specialist.

Distal PIN syndrome (posterior interosseus nerve syndrome) refers to entrapment of a motor branch of the radial nerve up the forearm near the lateral epicondyle. Entrapment is by muscles used in rotating the forearm or wrist. It is not common in keyboard work, but when it occurs it is likely related to the fact that the standard keyboard requires a palms-down (forearm rotated) attitude, while finger-extensor muscles (located on top of the rotation muscles) are rapid-firing for long periods of time.

The ulnar nerve travels down the inside of the arm and passes through several points of possible compression. It can be compressed where it passes over the elbow bone (ulnar bone), for example, by chronically leaning on the inside elbow bone. This cuts off significant blood flow and produces nerve compression.

Cubital tunnel syndrome refers to entrapment of the ulnar nerve at the cubital tunnel on the inside of the elbow. Computer workers who have their elbows bent at right angles most of the time are disposed to this condition.

The ulnar nerve passes through another tunnel, Guyon's Tunnel, in the wrist near the carpal tunnel. Working with the wrist constantly bent up and out is associated with this disorder.

Postural thoracic outlet syndrome (no. 5) affects the nerves and blood vessels that go to the arms as they pass through a narrow space (outlet) between the top rib and the collar bone. Postures, not uncommon in keyboard work, such as hunched shoulders, with arms close to the sides, or working with arms lifted and in front of you, can put pressure on the nerves and cause pain, tingling, numbness, and muscle weakness along the conduction paths of these nerves. The restriction of blood flow to arm tendons, ligaments, and muscles can produce chronically tired arms. Other conditions, such as overdeveloped or sagging muscles can dispose to TOS. Some cases of TOS are initially misdiagnosed as carpal tunnel syndrome.

There are a few more upper extremity disorders, but enough information has been provided to give the general character of these problems. In general, they involve wear and tear on tendons and tendon sheaths. The particular disorder is defined by the location of the damage. In some places, where tendons are located near nerves, swollen tissue can compress the nerve and lead to serious pain and disability if the swelling is allowed to continue. Knowing the general character of these disorders, the reader can easily understand how it is possible to have more than one disorder at a time. For example, the presence of cubital tunnel syndrome and Guyon's canal syndrome at the same time is called a "double crush." The expression "multiple crushes" is used to describe the presence of two or more syndromes.

Diagnosis of disorders is not a simple matter of knowing where the pain is. The tendon and nerve disorders are not always easy to distinguish. There is a painful disorder of the sympathetic nervous system, reflex sympathetic disorder (RSD), which can develop if other disorders are not treated. It is not always easy to distinguish RSD from TOS or one of the tunnel or tendon syndromes. If not correctly diagnosed and treated within six months, RSD pain can become severe and chronic. There are unrelated disorders with some of the same pain trigger points as CTDs—fibro-myalgia, for example. Tumors, Parkinsonism, multiple sclerosis, arthritis, and others can be confused with CTDs. Recently, Dr. David M. Glick reported that most patients presenting CTS symptoms (tingling, numbness, or pain in wrist and fingers) suffer from compression or irritation of a nerve in the cervical region of the spine.[13] The reader can understand why diagnosis is best left to a specialist. The specialist does not have to be a surgeon. In fact, a recommendation for surgery should be followed by a second expert opinion, because rest and job activity changes often lead to recovery.

The label "cumulative trauma disorder" carries with it the pre-diagnosis that a given syndrome is due to repetitive actions. At a two-day seminar on Cumulative Trauma Disorders of the Upper Extremity[14] sponsored by the American Association for Hand Surgery, several of the presenting hand-reconstruction surgeons expressed the opinion that CTDs are more often caused by medical conditions (arthritis, for example) than by repetitive and stressful jobs. They also expressed the opinion that the workers' compensation system is largely responsible for the recent flood of CTD patients, because workers are getting paid to complain. The opinion was expressed that workers complain about pain too much, and should be more willing to endure pain and difficult jobs.

Orthopedic surgeons exhibited a broader view of the issues. This difference in opinion about patient complaints and repetitive work may reflect differences in the training of orthopedic and reconstruction surgeons. After medical school, reconstruction surgeons specialize in learning how to cut and repair broken hands. In addition to hand surgery, orthopedic surgeons learn more about how joints, muscles, and tendons work and how they can be abused. They also get some training in occupational medicine or physical rehabilitation medicine.

Reconstruction surgeons do not have training in occupational issues and problems. They are accustomed to repairing hands damaged in auto accidents, or crushed by presses, where the damage is obvious. When presented with a hand that does not have obvious damage, and when the complaint is of pain, their skepticism is predictable. Consider such predisposition when weighing opinions. The conservative constellation of reconstructive surgeons' opinion may

13 Reported in *CTD News*, September 1993, 2(8), p. 8.

14 From a seminar, "Cumulative Trauma Disorders of the Upper Extremity," 1994, American Association of Hand Surgeons, August 12-13, Bloomington, MN.

constitute one side of a controversy for a few years. The other side will be argued by researchers who have done field research and worked on-the-job with workers.

Barbara Silverstein of OSHA, and Tom Hales of NIOSH, have this kind of experience. My experience has included watching CTD symptoms develop in repetitive, stressful jobs and improve over the weekend and during vacations. Some companies (Clorox, for example) have virtually eliminated CTD by using frequent job rotation. Many workers, supervisors, and hand therapists have this kind of experience which attests to the work-relatedness of the CTDs. Other writers and specialists (Pascarelli and Pinski, for example) have similar backgrounds. More formal studies on the effects of job repetition, rate rotation, length of exposure, and recovery after rest need to be published in the public arena. Meanwhile, we must acknowledge the controversy because it can present problems for a business that is trying to deal effectively with worker injury.

The hard-nosed surgeon or physician is inclined to minimize the patient's complaints of pain and work conditions and return them as soon as possible to the same, unmodified job after surgery or minimal treatment. Such medical professionals are disinclined, when filling out required forms, to attribute pain to injury, or injury to work conditions. Yet without firsthand knowledge of the patient's job or injury development the surgeon is simply in no position to decide that an injury (which could come from an occupational or a medical condition, or both) is not due, in some measure, to occupational factors. If the physician or surgeon also frequently minimizes patients' reports of pain as "complaining" or considers it something they should simply live with, you as a patient or employer had better get a second opinion.

There are some physicians and surgeons who tend to view patients as manipulative complainers, and consider their reports of pain as phony or exaggerated. They characteristically minimize and undermedicate for patient pain.[15, 16] As a cost-conscious

15 L. M. McCracken, et al., *Behavior Research and Therapy*, 1993, September 31 (7): 647-652.

16 N. H. Hendler, et al., "Overlooked Physical Diagnoses in Chronic Pain Patients Involved in Litigation," *Psychosomatics*, 1993, November/December: 34(6): 494-501.

businessperson, you may be tempted to believe such an opinion. However, you had better follow up on the patients who are returned to their same unmodified jobs, because untreated pain and injury gets worse and becomes *very* expensive to deal with. When having workers examined for possible injury and treatment it may be wise to have an orthopedic surgeon and/or a physician from medical specialties of occupational medicine or physical medicine and rehabilitation involved in the loop and responsible for evaluating the worker's job. Do not rely on a reconstructive surgeon for that.

⇨ The disabled worker

The space limitations for this section of this book prevent a complete, thorough presentation of specific applications for disabled workers. Fortunately this information is readily available from other sources, which are referenced in the footnotes at the bottom of the page they are mentioned throughout the chapter.

It is important to become acquainted with enabling possibilities because it is important that the handicapped be able to work. Another reason to learn about the federal Americans with Disabilities Act (ADA), as well as enabling possibilities, is that computer workers injured by CTD are using the provisions of ADA to legally force employers to make the accommodations necessary to return them to work.

Here is a brief description of the ADA. As of July 1994, the Act applies to employers of fifteen or more workers. It applies to all businesses and organizations, whether they are commercial enterprises or not. This includes employment agencies, labor organizations, state and local government.

The Act indicates conditions for hiring, promoting, offering health care, termination, making facilities accessible, and providing accommodations that enable employment. It also provides some consideration of the cost of making the accommodations. For example it requires that architectural and communication barriers be removed in existing facilities where the means for such removal are "readily available," and the needs of the disabled can be accommodated, "unless doing so would impose an undue hardship."

To help small businesses make physical accommodations, Congress provides a tax credit for businesses with fewer than 30 full-time employees. The business pays no more than $250 of the accommodation cost. The employer can get a 50 percent tax credit on costs over $250, up to $5,000 of actual cost. Costs above $5,000 qualify for a tax deduction of up to $15,000. Businesses with more than 30 employees, or $1 million in gross receipts, are limited to a $15,000 tax deduction. For more details read D. Fasman (1992),[17] Newell and Cairns (1993), and other sources listed here:

A Technical Assistance Manual of the Employment Provisions (Title 1) of the Americans with Disabilities Act, U.S. Equal Employment Opportunity commission, Resource Directory, 1992. A first copy is free. Call (800) 669-3362.

Foundation for Technology Access, 1128 Solano Ave., Albany, CA 94706, (800) 922-8111, (510) 528-0747.

Job Accommodation Network, 918 Chestnut Ridge Rd., Suite 1, P. O. Box 6080, Morgantown, WV 26506-6080, (800) 526-7234, or (304) 293-7186.

Madenta, 9411A-20 Ave., Edmonton, Alberta T6N 1E5 (800) 661-8406, (403) 428-5376. Provide software for the disabled—voice recognition, no-hands typing, limited body movement.

National Council on Disability, 800 Independence Ave. SW, Suite 814, Washington, DC 20581, (202) 293-5960.

Uniform Federal Accessibility Standards (1988) can be obtained from the National Council on Disability, or from the Department of Labor in your state.

Worldwide Disability Solutions Group, Apple Computer, 20525 Mariani Ave., Cupertino, CA 95014, (408) 924-7910.

17 Z. D. Fasman, 1992, *What Business Must Know about the ADA: 1992 Compliance Guide*, Washington, DC: U.S. Chamber of Commerce.

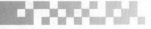

The Act covers the well-known disabilities (sight, hearing, loss of limbs) and medical conditions, including cancer, epilepsy, heart disease, contagious disease, psychiatric conditions, and learning disability. And now the courts are including occupational disabilities such as CTDs. The President's Committee on Employment for People with Disabilities has forced the Job Accommodation Network to provide free information to employers, rehabilitation specialists, and the disabled, or methods of accommodating the disabled. There is also a government funded effort in Canada at (800) 526-2262. Failure to comply can result in a civil lawsuit and/or fines up to $300,000.

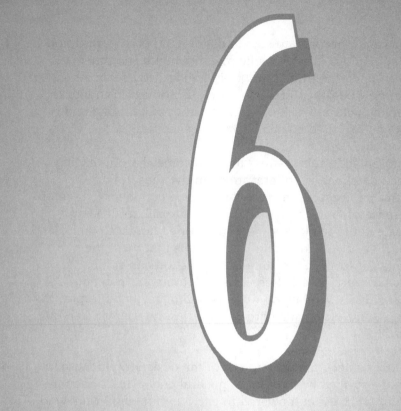

Computer workstation design standards & the OSHA general duty clause

CHAPTER 6

THE current approach to standards for computer workstation design employs many specific measurements and schematic drawings of an operator sitting upright in an idealized chair. As mentioned in previous chapters, this format is not very useful to a person grappling with the task of selecting from real seating and other components offered by persuasive salespeople.

Standards presented in this manner are also somewhat misleading. The term "standards" is often interpreted in the sense of "specifications" or "regulations" to which one *must* adhere. Taken in the weaker sense of "recommendation" they are still misleading, because they lead the workstation designer, or equipment purchaser, to think that their task is to obtain components that meet the measurements put forth in the standard. Selection can still be difficult, as when very different chairs are all touted as meeting ANSI/HFS standards. And many workers and managers interpret the bolt-upright posture of the standard operator as the way workers are supposed to sit.

A more useful and accurate description of the designer/purchaser's general duty is provided by the OSHA general duty clause. Section 5(a) states that OSHA is empowered to cite and fine employers who "fail to furnish each of their employees a place of employment free of recognized hazards causing or likely to cause death or serious physical harm." This general duty applies to *each and every* person in our place of work, including disabled workers, not only to the estimated 95 percent of the public as suggested by the measures provided by the ANSI/HFS standard.

Given the general duty to provide a workplace free of hazards to workers, the recommendations for safe (ergonomic) workplace design presented in the chapters dealing with health and safety-related issues should be interpreted as applying to each worker. The general-duty approach to standards has interesting complications regarding claims by some equipment manufacturers. For example, it is no longer possible for a chair manufacturer to say that their product meets the standard. If the employer's duty is to find the chair, or seating arrangement, that best meets the needs for each individual, then a given chair will meet the standard for some individuals but not for others. The employer meets the duty only by considering the needs of each worker, and that means considering more than a single one-size-fits-all alternative.

The standards approach to safe workplace design may say of seating, for example, that chair height should be variable from 16 to 19 inches. The OSHA general-duty approach may say that the workers should be provided with chairs that permit sitting with feet on the floor, which could be a whole different requirement in some cases.

One method of documentation being used to support safe treatment of the public in legal actions is *hazard analysis*. In the hazard-analysis procedure for a given product or a given worker, potential hazards are anticipated and documented. Worker participation is required in this effort. Actions taken to minimize or eliminate the hazards from the individual's workstation are recorded in the hazard-analysis folder for that individual, along with action taken and reasons for not dealing with some of them. These reasons can be used later as documentation of the employer's responsible action toward providing a safe workplace for each individual in case there is any question.

It should be noted about the ANSI/HFS standards that they are not at all like laws or regulations. They were put together primarily by representatives from business and industry, along with a few university professors. Worker groups were not prominently represented. They are an excellent source of general human factors information. However, voluntary standards organizations sponsored by corporations, such as ANSI and UL, have on occasion been criticized as representing mainly business interests (Meier 1991). Courts generally regard a voluntary standard, such as ANSI or UL, as a minimum criterion of corporate concern for safety, and not a criterion of safe design or safe conditions.

ANSI/HFS 100 (1988) neglected to address important aspects of VDT workstation design for health and safety. It did not address working conditions such as workload and work pace, work surges, fear about job security, work pace monitoring, all of which increase CTD symptom rates. It also ignored possible VDU radiation hazards (see Chapter 8) and vision problems.

OSHA standards are viewed in the same vein by civil courts. The main use of a standard such as ANSI/HFS 100 (1988), or any similar successor, would seem to be as advice on how to design a chair or work surface that will fit about 95 percent of workers. Employers with paid-up workers' compensation premiums have no legal obligation to follow it. But you still have to watch out for OSHA. They have even cited and heavily fined their own offices.[1]

More active participation of government agencies (the Commerce Department) and major worker groups (e.g., communication workers) would make future versions of ANSI/HFS more useful to employers looking for guidance in establishing safe working conditions. OSHA regulations do have the status of law because they are enforceable. Since OSHA will be coming out in a few months with more specific regulations, the general-duty approach to safe and healthy workplace design is worth exploring at this time.

Summary of health & safety & related issues

Here are some suggestions for a list of specific duties regarding the health and safety of VDT and computer workers, who do their work from a seated position.

➤ VDT operators should be provided with chairs that have adjustable lumbar (pelvic) support. The worker should also be provided a means for using that support whether sitting upright or leaning back. Pelvis pocket, back distance, and seat-pan depth could be among the considerations here.

➤ Operators should be provided with chairs that have shoulder-high backs and moving pans that permit work from a reclined position (120° or more), or from more upright postures including a forward tilt of 8 to 10 degrees.

---

1 "OSHA office is cited for unsafe working conditions," Minneapolis *Star Tribune*, April 28, 1994.

➤ Chair arms should be wide enough to prevent wobble and slide, and soft enough to prevent uncomfortable pressure on the elbow and soft tissues, such as the ulnar nerve, passing around the elbow. They should support the forearm and not contact the elbow.

➤ The chair arm should be long enough to support forearms, and adjustable for distance from the worker to help the worker attain a neutral wrist position for keyboard activity. The operator should not have to use shoulder and neck muscles to hold arms and hands in a neutral position.

➤ Keyboard and VDU placement and adjustability should permit working from a variety of reclining, upright, or forward postures.

➤ Keyboard slope or design should not require wrist extension (up, a non-neutral wrist position) or wrist deviation (sideways) for operation. Foam wrist pads should be used to increase wrist comfort and help attain a nonextended wrist position. They should support the heel of the hand rather than the wrist.

➤ Ancillary input devices (a mouse or a ball, for example) should be located nearby and on the same level as the keyboard.

➤ Operators should get up out of the seated posture and walk or engage in other locomotor-intensive activities for at least five minutes every hour.

➤ The VDU monitor should be movable forward and back, and tiltable up-down and side-to-side, to accommodate posture variation and lighting conditions that cause visual discomfort.

➤ Various accessories, such as copy holders, mouse pads, and footrests should be provided as needed.

➤ Operators should be actively encouraged to report any pain or discomfort associated with work conditions—posture, vision, work requirements, or any other factors.

Most likely, OSHA duties will be specified for video monitors relating to contrast, resolution, and radiation limits. One additional, much-needed duty would deal with daily limits on keystroking. In 1985 the Japanese set a limit of 300 minutes per day, with a rest break every hour. I inquired of OSHA officials working on the ergonomic standards and was told that there will most likely not be specific limits set on keystrokes. This is unfortunate, because business and workers both need guidance on limits that will reduce carpal tunnel disorder and the escalating costs associated with CTDs. The research needed to determine these limits could be provided by OSHA through NIOSH.

Lacking this information, some assistance in dealing with CTD frequency and cost could be provided by regulating the use of electronic monitoring of keystrokes, which is frequently used to set and control work requirements. Frontline managers, as well as workers, want to know how much is too much and want assistance in drawing the line. Companies want to control workers' compensation costs and prevent employee injury. Reasonable limits would be helpful in achieving both of these goals.

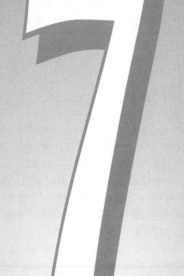

Are government regulation, law, & workers' compensation bad for business?

ALL cumulative traumas, or repetitive strain injuries, are covered by workers' compensation legislation in all states. Managers and workers should both have some knowledge of these laws.

Civil liability

British and American legal systems are similar for obvious reasons. To understand workers' compensation laws we must know the two kinds of laws in the British-American systems, statutes and common law. Statutes (codes) are laid down by the highest authority in a country, by royal decree or by a legislative body. Well-known codes in history have been those associated with Hammurabi, Rome (the Twelve Tables), Justinian, and Napoleon.

The code of Hammurabi is known for the "eye for an eye" principle. To prevent vengeful action between families, injury of one person by another was punished regardless whether it was accidental or intentional.

English common law evolved after 1100 A.D., when judges started keeping track of prior decisions in similar cases and using these as aids in making their own decisions. At this time and for 300 years more, the only consideration for *accidental* as opposed to *intentional* injury to another was given at royal discretion in the form of a pardon, usually depending on whether the defendant had placated the victim's family. After 1400 A.D., placation came most often in the form of money, which meant you could get off more readily if you were wealthy.

During the 17th and 18th centuries, common law decisions by the civil courts began to distinguish between intentional and unintentional injury, and a common person could be excused for unintentionally injuring another; for example, by accidentally firing a gun. However, the defendant would have to prove his innocence. Some accidents still had to be compensated for. Innkeepers, common carriers, or other places for operations of commerce might have to compensate victims for loss or injury on the premises, for either of two reasons.

First, if the proprietors were found negligent in observing a duty to try to prevent such accidents; and second, if they simply failed to prevent the accident. The latter circumstance developed out of the courts' concern over restoring the means to survive or thrive of damaged and suffering victims, and is called *strict liability*.

You can understand the latter option as the concern of the court trying to deal humanely with a newly disabled worker, or a new widow and children, with no support available. These sentiments, and the strict liability option, disappeared in both Britain and the United States when the industrial revolution shifted into high gear. One of the most interesting legal developments prior to the industrial revolution was the description of civil social behavior as involving enforceable duties on the part of each of us to help protect and support others in our country.

Since common law depends on precedent rather than code, it is more easily influenced by mood and sentiment at the time of litigation than are statute decisions. With the exploitation of steam engine power in locomotives, ships, mining, automobiles, and farm machinery, a general enthusiasm for power and industrial progress rapidly developed. This appeared in 19th and 20th century civil courtrooms as a reluctance to impede industry by imposing costly or time-consuming safety requirements or penalties. The argument was generally accepted that hazardous work and low pay were necessary for industrial development. The plaintiff had to prove not only negligence or intent to violate civil duty to provide safe work conditions, but that the dangers were *unreasonably* hazardous as well.

The socially uncontrolled entrepreneurial initiative that led to America's leap into world preeminence as an industrial power in the last third of the 19th century was accomplished by a ruthless spirit of competition that left little room for concern about the welfare or working conditions of those at the bottom (Weinstein 1967). This is consistent with the total absence of any reference to employee health, pain, or other work-related problems in the turn-of-the-century office texts (Galloway 1919; Leffingwell 1917) we have referenced in previous chapters. An eerie era.

The courts helped the industrial cause as much as possible by establishing precedents that made it virtually impossible for an injured worker to sue an employer in civil court with any success. For example:

> **Contributory negligence** Even the slightest lack of ordinary care by the worker barred recovery. If the employee contributed even 1 percent, and the employer 99 percent toward an injury, recovery was barred.

> **Fellow servant rule** If the accident was caused by the negligence of a co-worker, the employer was not liable.

> **Assumption of risk** The employee had the option of not working for a given employer. If he took the work he assumed the risks involved.

> **Rule of privaty** This rule was taken from contract law. Privaty is the relationship between buyer and seller. One cannot sue for injury by equipment unless one bought the equipment from the seller. Thus, injured workers could not sue their employer or equipment seller for defective equipment because they did not purchase the equipment from either party.

The Fourteenth Amendment to the Constitution was cleverly interpreted to prevent injured employees from recovering damages from employers. The amendment had been passed to establish constitutional rights for freed Negroes and says, in part, that states shall not pass laws that violate ". . . the liberty of the individual in adopting or pursuing such calling as he may choose." Employers successfully argued that occupational regulations would interfere with the rights of the individual to take any job for which he was willing to assume the risk.

There were quite a few additional obstacles in the way of recovery through civil court proceedings; for example, the lack of funds to pay medical bills and living expenses during the litigation. Cases took anywhere from six months to six years for resolution. The injured worker had justifiable fears of being terminated for bringing suit, and co-workers who knew of the employer's negligence refused to testify for fear of being fired themselves. If the ruling was favorable for the injured worker, the lawyers got most of the award.

In sum, these barriers were pretty effective. Estimates have it that, prior to 1910, no more than 15 percent of injured workers ever recovered damages through common law, even though 70 percent of such injuries were related to working conditions or employer negligence (Rosenblum 1973). Workers' compensation laws in the United States were delayed for decades after similar legislation was passed in Prussia, Czarist Russia, Austria, Germany, and Great Britain.

Oddly, early attempts to formulate compensation legislation in this country were opposed by unions (Weinstein 1967, p. 160). They thought that state provision of benefits and pensions for injury victims would reduce worker loyalty to unions. Instead, they lobbied for legislation that would reduce the employer defenses, previously mentioned, that effectively prevented recovery in civil court. They thought, probably correctly, that civil court awards would be much more generous than a compensation schedule. But by 1910 the unions had given up on changing common law and were supporting workers' compensation legislation at the federal level.

Also oddly, in 1910, manufacturers, through the National Association of Manufacturers, endorsed a proposal for workers' compensation legislation (statutes). They realized that compensation was coming in some form and thought that private insurance-company plans and self-funded plans would be too expensive for small manufacturers.

With labor and industry more or less supporting legislative action, and unions gaining strength, a general inclination toward action was provided by a series of catastrophic boiler explosions and fires on steamboats and locomotives. In 1833 Andrew Jackson had asked Congress for legislation to deal with the "criminal negligence" relating to safety on boats. The infamous Triangle Shirtwaist Factory fire in 1911, in which 146 workers died because employers had reduced the size of exits, helped obtain passage of federal workers' compensation laws. President Theodore Roosevelt in 1908 declared "an outrage" the lot of the disabled worker and his family. He was influential in the 1908 passage of a compensation law for coal miners in Montana.

In general, the courts regarded worker compensation as radical and revolutionary. Roosevelt's reaction to a New York Court of Appeals decision in 1911, *Ives v. South Buffalo Railway Co.*, got the attention of the courts and hurried passage of compensation legislation. In 1910, New York had become the first state to adopt a general compulsory workers' compensation law. But in 1911 the Appeals Court ruled that the New York law was unconstitutional on the grounds of deprivation of property without due process of law (i.e., imposition of liability without finding fault). Roosevelt was so angry that he proposed the passage of laws to allow the recall of judicial decisions. At that point the courts suddenly became more supportive of compensation.

In 1917, the U.S. Supreme Court ruled that compulsory compensation laws were constitutional. Compensation laws followed piecemeal in each of the states, starting with Wisconsin in 1911. Of the original 48 states, the last adopting state was Mississippi in 1948. The District of Columbia, Guam, Puerto Rico, American Samoa, the U.S. Virgin Islands, and both Alaska and Hawaii also have workers' compensation laws. They all differ in coverage and benefits, as can be seen in Tables I and II in the appendix to this book.

There is a sense in which workers' compensation legislation arrived just in time for industry in this country. Civil courts have now become more concerned with safety, and the contrived obstacles to injured-party recovery have been largely dropped. In fact the most humane of principles, strict liability, has made its way back into present-day civil courts. By this principle, the plaintiff is not required to establish negligence by the defendant in order to recover. However, negligence is still the primary justification for recovery in most injury suits. The injuries may be incurred by patrons in a place of commerce, or by users of products that were hazardous in design or manufacture. The public establishment of negligence and hefty punitive damage awards has been the major stimulus to improved safety in design of products and facilities. For example, who hasn't heard of the Ford Pinto case, or GM's sidesaddle gas tanks on certain trucks?

The same incentive to improve safety in the workplace does not occur under workers' compensation, because the employee recovers without establishing fault and is not allowed to sue the employer for negligence. There are no punitive damage awards, and a private insurance company makes the payments (i.e., buffers the cost). Also, the compensation levels are quite minimal; for example, a total disability award generally does not meet the poverty level for a family of four. In some states the compensation schedules are downright miserly. In Louisiana, for example, a temporary total disability receives only 28.42 percent of wages lost. The families of workers killed in an explosion at the Thiokol Chemical plant in Georgia a few years ago were compensated at $40 per week for 400 weeks, for a total of $16,000 per family (Hammer 1989). Obviously, other social support agencies, and the social security system, have to make up the difference. Not a bad deal for employers, when the alternative of a safety-minded civil court is considered.

There *are* conditions that expose employers to civil actions for workplace injury; for example, if the employer does not pay into the workers' compensation system or is late with a premium payment. If the employer fails to file required injury documentation they also become vulnerable (Rosenblum 1973).

⇨ Criminal liability

In general, workers' compensation and OSHA do not protect employers from criminal prosecutions. Do you remember reading about the *People v. Film Recovery* case, in which workers recovering silver from film negatives were poisoned by cyanide gas from the bubbling vats? The employers, who knew about the hazards but did not inform their workers, were sentenced to twenty-five-year prison terms and fined $24,000 each. The principle that employers remain open to criminal prosecution when they are responsible, deliberately or by negligence, for deaths or serious injury of employees, is being upheld in Supreme Courts throughout the U.S. (Larson 1988).

The lack of hazard deterrence in the workers' compensation system has allowed the continuation of dangerous working conditions. Catastrophes similar to the Triangle Shirtwaist Factory fire continue to occur. For example, consider the recent fire in a Hamlet, North

Carolina chicken-processing plant, where workers died because the employer had locked the escape exits.

The only effective deterrents to workplace injury have been strong unions and, more recently, the federal Occupational Safety and Health Act (OSHA) of 1970. Both the unions and OSHA administration revealed their weakness in the face of political pressure during the Reagan and Bush presidential years. But since then they have been showing a few signs of recovery, responding enough to encourage intense lobbying. OSHA has worked hard at reducing worker injury in meat-processing plants, and has been actively pursuing cumulative trauma in white-collar computer-work environments. They have cited and fined newspapers and telephone companies for hazardous computer-work conditions. Keyboard manufacturers are being sued in civil courts for producing hazardous products, although demanding work requirements are probably more culpable than the keyboards, per se.

Unions are starting to show more results in bargaining and striking for workplace safety. For example, the Teamsters recently prevented United Parcel from increasing the package-lifting limit for one person from 75 to 150 pounds. Had OSHA been on the ball it could have prevented that strike by citing United Parcel for exceeding OSHA lifting limits on most 75-pound lifts.

One advantage for business of a strong OSHA, besides lower medical and compensation costs, would be the reduction in frequency of wasteful strikes.

The case for some OSHA regulation can be underscored. For example, without enforced safety and health regulations there eventually will be publicity over worker abuse, if only by a few reckless or callous employers. Nevertheless, the embarrassment and costs of legislative reform will be borne across the entire spectrum of industry.

Look at a few of the consequences of public reaction to the fire that killed 56 workers in the Hamlet, North Carolina, chicken-processing plant of Imperial Food Products Company in 1991.

➤ The passage by the North Carolina legislature of twelve new laws that compel much closer scrutiny of workers' compensation rates and results of frequent safety inspections to define hazardous jobs.

➤ The installation of worker safety committees in companies with eleven or more employees occupied in hazardous jobs.

➤ The installation of a whistle-blower program in which employees who report, or threaten to report, unsafe conditions have job protection and the prospect of collecting triple damages if fired.

➤ The subjection of state agencies and government employers to the same regulations and penalties as private companies if they violate OSHA regulations.

➤ More frequent inspections as a result of 77 new Health and Safety inspectors being hired by the state.

➤ The loss of the next election by the anti-OSHA head of the North Carolina Department of Labor.

➤ The gaining of more influence in state parties by the AFL-CIO. At the federal level, legislation for federal takeover of all state-run OSHA programs was introduced. Federal OSHA conducted special investigations in all 23 states that run their own OSHA programs and in some that don't; Georgia, for example.

➤ The levying of six-digit fines.

➤ The requirement that federal OSHA must investigate the backlog of North Carolina's worker-health and safety complaints.

➤ The requirement that USDA inspectors must take training in worker health and safety, and report OSHA violations along with food processing problems.[1]

It's my perception that public reaction to CTDs, in white-collar as well as in blue-collar jobs, is growing to the extent that, as a direct result, strong reform will take place at the federal level sooner or

1 The News and Observer of Raleigh, NC was a valuable source of information on this incident.

111

later. If later, then we take the risk of allowing it to occur as an overreaction to publicized employee abuse by a small number of employers. It would be much better for business if needed regulation could be formulated in a voluntary climate of balancing the needs of both labor and business rather than a contest of political clout. And it would be much better if OSHA did a good job of inspecting and enforcing those regulations with its current policy of warnings and gentle, non-punitive fines. One reason the CTD issue is not going to run out of publicity steam is that media workers themselves are among those having the problems.

How to control workers' compensation costs

Workers' compensation costs represent a significant portion of payroll; five to ten percent for most businesses. In the past this expense has been fatalistically accepted as an unavoidable cost of doing business, and the only action taken was that of making insurance-premium payments.

With rising medical costs, rising workers' compensation costs are stimulating a greater variety of actions. For example:

> ➤ Intense lobbying is now underway to reduce employer contributions and compensation schedules. Employers with some knowledge of the history of worker compensation may have a sense that, right now, workers compensation is a better deal for employers than it is for employees. If compensation becomes generally publicized as inadequate, and history repeats, civil courts will be enlisted again to settle claims, and federal legislation will be passed. Strict liability is now an operating principle of civil courts, and large punitive awards are employed to induce improvements in worker safety. Monetary disincentives associated with OSHA citations are negligible by comparison.

> To some extent, employer lobbying can help control potential compensation rate increases. Threatening to move or expand operations in another state or country with lower compensation

rates continues to be effective, along with portraying the American business climate as near death in the face of compensation costs. Federal law can be developed to reform civil (that is, "common") law.

➤ Quite a few cases involving heavy compensation costs have occurred at smaller companies, where only two or three disabilities can take the company below profitability. OSHA standards could help protect companies not in the workers' compensation system from negligence lawsuits. Businesses who are not taking active steps, such as those described below, may be allowing their costs to escalate.

➤ Companies in two-thirds of the states could benefit from effective lobbying at the state level for a reduction in employer contribution when social security disability benefits kick in. Another offset can be obtained in some states when unemployment benefits kick in.

Note that there are a few states in which a disincentive to go back to work can occur when disabled workers receive benefits from three sources that amount to more than the original wage—workers' compensation, social security, and unemployment insurance. A few publicized cases like this can give the entire workers' compensation system a bad name.

Tables I and II in the appendix provide some information on benefits and offsets offered in the states. Table II indicates state compensation for type and degree of disability.[2] Note the difference between states. The hand of a disabled Colorado employee, for example, is worth approximately $\frac{1}{20}$ the hand of a federal worker, or $\frac{1}{6}$ the hand of a Connecticut employee.

Publicity over inadequate compensation in some states, and the attending poverty and misery, could lead to a public outcry and reform of compensation rates for all states. Lobbying for legislation that will provide more nearly equivalent compensation in all states could, if effective, help keep costs down in most states and could forestall federal takeover of worker compensation.

2 A complete description of workers' compensation award schedules and exceptions can be found in *Analysis of Workers' Compensation Laws*, Washington, DC: U.S. Chamber of Commerce. A new edition comes out every year.

> Companies have an option for self-insurance in most states.

> Reducing work-related injuries through workstation and work schedule changes has been an effective way to control payout costs.

Many published case histories document a significant reduction in workers' compensation and other medical costs after the instituting of improvements in computer workstation ergonomics (Herbert 1993; Sauter, Dainoff, and Smith 1990). One needs training and experience, however, in making these changes. Automating or outsourcing computer-intensive work is recommended.[3] Some useful information about computer workstation hazards can be obtained from OSHA,[4] union-sponsored programs,[5] or business-sponsored sources.[6] The latter can be a bit expensive.

> Disputing the work-related character of an accident or disorder is often successful, because employees may engage in other activities that cause the problem. For example, an employee may run a word-processing or programming business during evenings or weekends. Knitting or guitar-playing may be intense avocations. The relation of these activities to work activities, and to potential cumulative trauma, should be indicated to the worker and noted in his hazard-analysis record.

The most frequent claim is hearing loss, although some loss occurs naturally with age. Compensation is not allowed if the injured worker was intoxicated or started a fight, or if he was using company equipment (such as the machine shop) for personal work. Driving to and from work is not covered unless the employer provides the transportation, or asks the employee to report in or leave at a time or place that differs from the

---

3 However, there are cases in progress in which an attempt is being made to establish the principle that liability for injury is not outsourced along with the work.

4 You can access OSHA and NIOSH resources by first contacting your state OSHA office.

5 For example, two resources with good information are: (a) Labor Occupational Health Program (LOHP), School of Public Health, University of California at Berkeley, California 94720, 415-642-5507. (b) 9 to 5, National Association of Working Women, National Office, 614 Superior Ave. NW, Cleveland, OH 44113, 216-566-9308.

6 Center for Office Technology, 1800 N. Kent St, Suite 1160, Rosslyn, VA 22209, 703-276-1174.

usual, or if the employee is taking work home. Notably, illegal employees such as minors or aliens are, in some states, awarded from one to three times the compensation of a legal employee.

➤ Checking for dishonesty can help. Most claimants are honest and will help if asked. For example, questionable medical bills can be shown to the injured worker. The worker will tell you if the billed visit, procedure, or medication never took place.

Occasional false claims by employees do surface. Experienced case-management personnel can often pick out cases worth investigating. Some clues: injuries precede expected plant closings; a claimant may receive mail at a post office box; a claimant will not divulge his home address and does not answer his home telephone; he has frequent and large compensation claims; the claimant moves out-of-state.

I've recently discussed the issue of false claims with retired United Parcel management, who found it beneficial to investigate some claims. This may not be the case for computer-related cases in other occupations. It deserves checking.

➤ Case management. Companies are finding that taking an active role in each case can reduce costs. Some elements of an effective management system have been pretty well established.

• Cases are two times more expensive when the claimant hires a lawyer. Often, the lawyer is hired simply to explain the workers' compensation system and the claimant's rights, and to find out what to do next. The Walt Disney Company in Burbank, California, reduced the frequency of litigated claims from more than 65 percent in 1974 to less than 10 percent currently by publishing a booklet entitled *Everything You Wanted to Know About Workers' Comp But Were Afraid to Ask*. A toll-free number was included for answering questions.

• Maintaining contact with the employee can also help. A conversation between a company representative and the injured worker should take place within twenty-four hours. The conversation should be supportive and should provide information on procedure, benefits, and treatment providers. Information communicated during the call can remove the need for paperwork the employee usually fills out. Supportive and informative conversation between the case manager (preferably the same one) and the worker should take place every few days. The employee should know that the company is interested in his/her return as soon as possible. One study reported that injured workers who heard from their employers soon after the injury returned to work 20 percent sooner than those not contacted.[7]

➤ The operating principle stressed in this relationship, reciprocation of sentiment, is the same one involved in constructive working relationships generally, and deserves repeating. People care about people who care about them, and dislike people who dislike or don't care about them. People will care for your company, and work for you (I mean, really *work*) if they can see that you genuinely do care about them. This principle really does operate at the personal level and is a major motivating force in effective pupil performance in school as well as in a company. Fail to communicate, or communicate only through an officious third-party insurance provider, and you may turn a short-term disability into one of those expensive long-term ones. An absence can become a dropout.

States that allow workers to choose their physician tend to have lower workers' compensation costs (Davisson 1994). This may have something to do with convincing the worker that his health and rehabilitation is an important concern for the company.

➤ Three-way communications between company, doctor, and employee is important. There should be discussion prior to treatment so that the treatment can be explained and employer questions can be answered at that time. Employer reservations expressed *after* treatment create a bad impression of the company. In business jargon this may be called an up-front utilization review. Often a doctor will need information about the kind of work that a returning employee is going to return to before deciding if return to work is possible. Without that

---

7 Cited by M. R. Costigan, "Employee Empowerment," *Business Insurance*, September 16, 1991, p. 57.

information a doctor can be reluctant to send a worker back to the company.

➤ Early return to work is the best way to get a claim off the books. It doesn't take a great deal of creativity to establish transitional work that doesn't reactivate injuries. The transition period can be used for education. For example, you may need a few more trained, experienced workers to implement active, money-saving programs in workers' compensation liaison and administration, safety, early detection of CTD symptoms, re-engineering of injury-prone work to suggest just a few possibilities.

➤ Assist the injured worker in claiming social security disability benefits. These can help reduce employer liability in sixteen states: Alaska, California, Colorado, Florida, Louisiana, Michigan, Minnesota, Montana, New Hampshire, New Jersey, New York, North Dakota, Oregon, Utah, Washington, and Wisconsin. Saskatchewan and six other Canadian provinces have similar policies.

A word of caution. These are times of intense business lobbying against prospective OSHA legislation at state and federal levels, and for cuts in employer contributions to workers' compensation benefits.

If history serves, there may be more to fear from winning these battles than from not winning. The workers' compensation system protects employers in many ways. There are *many* active steps companies can take to reduce their costs, without trying to lower already-low benefit schedules. Small companies need special assistance in compensating their workers.

Benefits could be lowered to the point at which proposed federal legislation to federalize compensation will occur as an overreaction to publicized abuse and impoverishment of injured workers in one or more of the low-compensation, anti-labor states. Examples of this process are available.

Proposals for OSHA regulation are considerate of business in their present form. In fact, the proposal for a California OSHA ergonomics standard does not provide enough guidance and protection for employers, because it does not specify limits for keyboard use. Research-based limits would help reduce injury rates and compensation costs.

Current anti-regulation lobbying in the name of business has the dimensions of a mindless phobia. Thirty-four states would rather pay double compensation than offset for social security and, just possibly, take a chance on awakening the slumbering federal bear.

Let us be certain that we know what we are doing when we take a position on OSHA regulation or workers' compensation. Let us be sure that the lobbyists have not found a way to milk industry by using alarmism about regulation of any kind, which can then send them rushing, like high-priced fire departments, to put out the fire they themselves created.

Unions engage in their own kinds of mindless phobia. Attempts to make work safer or more efficient are often resisted if there will be a change in job definition, seniority prerogatives, or workforce reductions. OSHA safety regulations can assist employers in defining hazardous jobs and re-engineering the work (Larson 1988).

If you are a manager in the federal Social Security administration, or the General Accounting Office, I have a couple of ideas on how you can cut some of your disability expenses. An Associated Press release, appearing in the *Minneapolis Star Tribune* for March 11, 1994, described how only one percent of all disability recipients ever give up their benefits because they have recovered. A 1980 law requires that the Social Security Administration conduct .4 to .5 million reviews every year of ill or injured workers receiving Social Security disability compensation. However, the agency has conducted fewer than .05 million reviews in the past three years, even though it saves $6 for every $1 spent doing the reviews. How do we get a recovered worker back to work, and off workers' compensation, when the SSA pays them to stay home?

Some of them might be able enough to do review work for the SSA, and the SSA does need more workers.

One big reason why there is little federal oversight, and so much overlooking on Social Security disability, is that it's not the reviewer's money that is being spent, it's *ours*, as private companies and private individuals. The SSA employees are spending somebody else's money, so why bother checking?

Patten recently listened to a program on public radio about a naturalized citizen from Jordan who, though well off running his dry-cleaning business, had duped a doctor into supporting his social security claim for mental-illness disability. His friends were doing it, too. Why? Because his wife wanted a Mercedes. The justification? America is the land of opportunity, and doesn't everybody cheat a little bit—on their taxes, for example? The SSA will even pay nonworkers $400 to $600 a month for acquiring a drug-habit disability. The payments, which can be used to buy drugs, continue as long as habit continues. Why stop? They don't.

Maybe it would pay if we did more checking on our own company's disability recipients. The SSA might be interested in our findings. The existence of little or no oversight of federal disability expenditures makes it tough on companies who want to get their workers off disability and back to productive work.

In general, the taxing and spending prerogatives of the U.S. government are truly amazing. They can spend as much as they want; there is no effective budget because, if they want more, they simply borrow more and charge it to us through bonds and bills, or take it from social security, or charge us more taxes. They have all our credit cards and they are running them up, and we're paying an awful lot of interest. Wouldn't it be a whole lot easier if you could run your business this way? As private individuals and companies, we have to face the reality of real budgets, which involve limited funds and spending our own money.

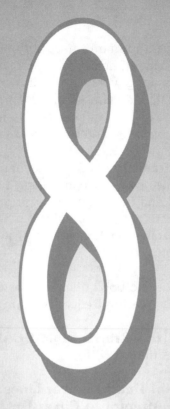

Is radiation from video display units a hazard?

CHAPTER 8

RADIATION is an important topic, not only because it relates to computer workstation health and safety but also because there is a growing concern among workers, and in worker unions, over possible hazards of VDU radiation. Managers and supervisors will need some grasp of the history and current status of the issues to deal credibly with worker concerns, and to provide safe VDU workstations.

The issue of health hazards from electromagnetic fields (EMF) is a major controversy right now. The controversy has been developing in the past fifteen years, and there is currently a great deal of populist agitation for government action (Nye 1994), as well as business lobbying against government action. All of this is taking place largely behind the media stage.

Nevertheless, headlines and book titles such as the following have been appearing with increasing frequency during the 80s:

(headline) **STUDY LINKS RISKS OF MISCARRIAGE TO HEAVY VDT USE** (Altman 1988)

(book title) **Currents of Death: Power Lines, Computer Terminals, and the Attempt to Cover Up Their Threat to Your Health** (Brodeur 1989)

Despite occasional blurbs like these, a pretty tight lid has been kept on widespread public reaction by the combined work of our federal government, business lobbying, a cool media, and a genuine lack of information. This has kept the legal front fairly quiet, despite juicy tort litigation prospects. "The omnipresence of EMF(s) in our daily lives suggests that this new litigation has the potential to open up a legal abyss that would dwarf the ones created by asbestos" (Krieger 1994).

Articles about EMF hazards have discussed VDUs in combination with EMF from power lines. Although EMF levels of the two are similar in some circumstances, it is advisable to separate power line problems from VDU issues as much as possible, for two reasons. First, the public has little control over power-line radiation, and so the potential level of fear is great. Second, there is some evidence for power lines hazards (e.g., A. Ahlbom, et al. 1993) and that controversy will be around for a long time, because reducing those hazards will be a prolonged, costly procedure.

Workers and managers have a good deal of potential control over VDU radiation, and radiation reduction is rapidly achievable at low expense. Thus, the VDU controversy will be discussed separately from the power line controversy.

⇨ VDU radiation

The typical cathode-ray tube (CRT) (Fig. 8-1) that is used in VDUs consists of an electron gun which shoots electrons into phosphor-dot bull's-eyes painted on the inside of the display surface. A "fly-back" transformer accelerates the electron beam toward the screen using a force of 15 to 25 kV. The phosphor dots glow when hit by the electron beam.

Figure 8-1

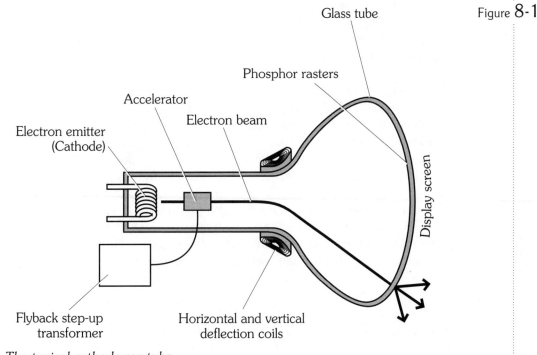

The typical cathode-ray tube.

The screen has rows of phosphor dots, called raster lines, that produce images with their afterglow as the electron beam is deflected up, down, and across the raster lines.

Movement of the electron beam across the screen is controlled by vertical and horizontal deflection coils mounted like a collar around the neck of the CRT. The coils produce magnetic fields that deflect the beam in a vertical or horizontal direction. The horizontal deflection coil is turned on and off fifteen thousand times each second to produce a horizontal scan rate of 15 kilohertz. This 15-kilohertz pulsing magnetic field is in the VLF (very-low-frequency) range of the radio frequency area of the electromagnetic spectrum. The vertical deflection coil is pulsed on and off only 60 times a second for a vertical scan rate of 60 Hertz. The 60-Hertz pulsing magnetic field of the vertical deflector coils falls in the extra-low-frequency (ELF) range of the radio frequency range. VDUs generally give higher ELF than VLF readings in the vicinity of the operator. With both deflection coils operating, the electron beam is actually deflected at an angle, from the lower left to the upper right corners of the screen, to produce the "sawtooth" scan pattern that will be mentioned if you read the articles cited in the bibliography that pertain to this chapter.

The CRT is a small particle accelerator, which produces "radioactive" (i.e., ionizing) radiation when the electrons smash into their targets. However, the weak ionizing radiation (gamma rays, x-rays, and some ultraviolet radiation) does not travel beyond the confines of the CRT and is not regarded as a health hazard. the CRT glass contains lead, which helps prevent the escape of ionizing radiation.

The pulsing invisible VLF and ELF magnetic (Fig. 8-2) fields do leave the CRT and can be detected surrounding the VDU. It is these fields, created by the vertical and horizontal deflection coils, that are the main issue of concern over VDU health hazards.

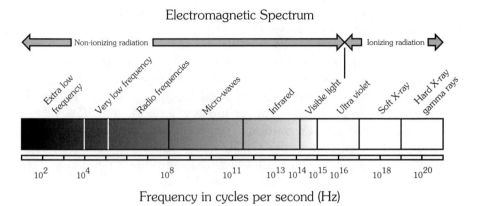

Electromagnetic Spectrum

Figure 8-2

The electromagnetic frequency spectrum.

Is VDU radiation a cause for concern?

This issue can be clarified by discriminating between two separate questions. First, is the *kind* of radiation that emanates from VDUs, mainly pulsed VLF and ELF, something to be concerned about? And second, if the *kind* is dangerous, is the *level* of pulsed VLF and ELF found around VDUs a cause for concern?

Despite the noise, dust, and confusion of the apparent controversy, the answer to the first question is a clear YES. The answer is clear because of the pragmatic, utilitarian aspect of scientific reasoning from evidence. The utility principle says in effect that, if you have much to lose and little to gain by drawing a conclusion or taking action based on evidence, then it is reasonable to be very cautious and require great certainty of outcome before doing it. Conversely, if you have little to lose and much to gain, then it is reasonable to draw a conclusion and take action on the basis of suggestive evidence, rather than to assume great risk through inaction while waiting years for "conclusive scientific evidence" to accumulate and pass scrutiny.

Given the principle of utility, question 1 becomes simply, "Is there any credible evidence that pulsed VLF and ELF might be harmful?"

Without doing an exhaustive review of the scientific literature, I've found several credible studies.

For example, researchers at the Institute of Occupational Health in Helsinki, Finland, have reported a much greater incidence of miscarriage for women who worked at VDUs giving off high levels of ELF and VLF (above 3 mG) than for those who worked at VDUs giving off lower levels of radiation. There was a greater miscarriage incidence if they worked at their VDU many hours per week (ten or more) than if they did VDU work fewer than ten hours per week (Lindbohm et al. 1992; Lindbohm et. al. 1993).

Duration of exposure to VLF and ELF during VDU work has been related to miscarriage incidence in several studies. For example, Goldhaber, Polen, and Hiatt (1988) studied 1,580 women who visited Kaiser Permanente obstetrics and gynecology clinics in the South Bay of San Francisco in 1981 and 1982. They reported that women who used VDUs more than 20 hours per week had an 80 percent greater risk of miscarriage than women who did comparable kinds of work but did not use VDUs. There was also a tendency to birth defects among offspring of the women having the greater risk of miscarriage.

The VDU radiation effects are not limited to miscarriage and birth defects. A relation of VDU use to brain tumors has been reported (Ryan 1992). Other studies show ELF and VLF effects on men as well as women.

This brief coverage of studies relating ELF and VLF from VDUs is not a thorough review of the published research on this topic. Only enough has been presented to establish the point that there is credible cause for concern about ELF and VLF from VDUs.

Subsequent research may establish the hazard as very minimal, or indicate that studies showing harmful effects are irreparably flawed. However, at present, it seems reasonable to conclude that ELF and VLF may have harmful effects.

Quite a few institutions are recognizing the possibility of electromagnetic hazards, as suggested by initial studies and surveys, and are taking the utilitarian approach of preventive and corrective actions as though the hazards did, in fact, exist. The Swedish government has made such a decision and has recommended the following limits (the Swedish MPR II limits)[1] for ELF and VLF for VDUs: A limit of 2.5 mG ELF measured 50 cm from the front of the VDU. The Swedish union TCO (Swedish Confederation of Professional Employees) has recommended a more stringent standard of 2 mG at 30 cm.

The MPR II and TCO limits are based on the desire to lower ELF and VLF as much as possible, given present technology. Dr. Yngve Hamnerius and his colleagues at Chalmers University of Technology in Göteborg, Sweden, say that the MPR II limits can be achieved for a factory cost of about $1.00 per VDU. The technology for this employs saddle-shaped compensation coils next to the horizontal and vertical deflection coils.[2]

In the United States, the National Foundation for Cancer Research (NFCR) is recommending the strict TCO limits. The New York City schools are requiring compliance with limits that are stricter than MPR II: ELF Limit: 2 mG at 30 cm; VLF Limit: 0.25 mG at 50 cm. They are giving preferential consideration to units meeting the TCO standards. In addition, the schools have asked for a minimum capital character height of 4.1 mm, because it permits students to keep a distance from the screen.[3]

The second question being considered in this chapter is whether ELF and VLF from VDUs is a cause for concern. The studies cited above suggest a yes answer. However, the more important question from the reader's point of view, is whether *your* VDU gives cause for concern. If you are concerned there are things you can do. You can check the ELF and VLF specifications for your unit. If these cannot be located you can contact the vendor or manufacturer. Either one of these may be willing to take measurements for you, or to recommend qualified personnel for the task.

1 The Swedish Board for Measurement and Testing; now named SWEDAC, the Swedish Board for Technical Accreditation.

2 *VDT News*, January/February, 1992.

3 Ibid.

If the reader is technically inclined, instruments for taking ELF and VLF measurements are available for purchase by the public. Check back issues of *VDT News* for instrument advertisements. Good instruments tend to be a bit expensive—over $200 by my guess. We have been using a Teslatronics model 70 that cost about $450.[4] We have calibrated it against some *very* expensive instruments and find the results to be extremely close.

There is a potential for abuse here with cheap, unreliable instruments and unqualified personnel, so take care. If you cannot obtain specifications or measurements for your unit you can be fairly sure of meeting MPR II standards by viewing your monitor from arm's length. Also, work at least four feet from the sides or back of a VDU.

Quite a few of the monitors meet MPR II standards even if they don't advertise it. Be sure to find out before you buy. *VDT News* publishes a list of companies that offer at least one VDU model that complies with MPR II limits.[5] Following is the most recent list available prior to publications.[6]

Low EMF Monitors

Apple Computer Inc.	(800) 776-2333
Applied Digital Data Systems, Inc.	(516) 342-7400
Compaq Computer Corp.	(800) 345-1518
Computer Lab International Inc.	(800) 727-5250
Cornerstone Imaging Inc.	(408) 435-8900
CTX International Inc.	(800) 282-2205
Dell Computer Corp.	(800) 289-3355
Digital Equipment Corp.	(800) 332-4636
E-Machines Inc.	(800) 344-7274
ETC Computer Inc.	(510) 226-6250

4 Teslatronics, 1310 Hollenbeck Ave., Suite C, Sunnyvale, CA 94087, 408-522-3770.

5 *VDT News: The Computer Health and Safety Report*, P. O. Box 1799, Grand Central Station, New York, NY 10163, 212-517-2802.

6 For an up-to-date list of monitors meeting MPR II and the more strict TCO standards, send one dollar to *VDT News*, address above.

Hewlett Packard Co.	(800) 752-0900
IBM Corporation	(800) 426-3333
IDEA Courier Inc.	(508) 663-6878
Matsushita Electric Corp.	(201) 348-7000
Mirror Technologies Inc.	(800) 654-5294
Mitsubishi Electronics America Inc.	(800) 843-2515
Mobius Technologies Inc.	(800) 523-7933
Nanao Corp.	(310) 325-5202
NEC Technologies Inc.	(617) 893-5700
NSA/Hitachi	(800) 388-8888
Optiquest Inc.	(800) 843-6784
Panasonic Office Automation	(800) 742-8086
Portrait Display Labs	(800) 858-7744
Qume Peripherals Inc.	(310) 802-8425
Radius Inc.	(800) 227-2795
Samtron Displays Inc.	(310) 802-8425
Seiko Instruments USA Inc.	(408) 922-5900
Sigma Designs	(800) 845-8086
Sony Corp. of America	(800) 352-7669
Tandberg Data Inc.	(800) 258-8285
ViewSonic	(800) 888-8583
Wyse Technology	(408) 473-1200

Source: *VDT News*, September/October 1993

One last word on limits. If your unit does not meet MPR II limits, please do not donate it to a school.

➪ The VDU radiation controversy

There is argument about the hazards of VDU radiation, with VDU manufacturers and government agencies minimizing or denying the hazard possibilities. It is not a big public controversy yet—at least, not in many areas of the United States. For example, I could not find a copy of Paul Brodeur's book, *Currents*, in any bookstore in the Minneapolis-St. Paul area of 2.5 million people. But then it's pretty hard to become a hotbed of anything when you're dealing with snow banks and wind chill. Thus, depending on location, a manager or supervisor who decides to ignore the utility aspect of reasoning and take the "I don't believe it" approach will probably be able to get away with doing nothing by citing some of the government or industry literature on the subject. Citations are available in the following paragraphs.

Brodeur, in his *New Yorker* article (1989), seems to paint the skeptical response of government and the "in denial" response of industry with a rather broad brush of cover-up and conspiracy. That is understandable from one who is writing with frustration and anger, and has the factual ducks pretty well lined up, but the unkindness is largely undue for the situation is very complex. Many factors are involved.

➤ Confusion about how to deal with skimpy, apparently inconsistent data.

➤ Customary scientific skepticism about anomalous findings for which there is no ready explanation, rather than utilitarian reasoning appropriate to hazard evaluation.

➤ Appeal to authority. August bodies of scientists from many famous universities have been assembled by government agencies to engage in the activities described directly above (for example, Oak Ridge Associated Universities in 1992). The Oak Ridge book contains excellent reviews of radiation effects on cells, glands, embryos, bone growth, cancer, and reproduction, which note definite ELF effects. The reviews are followed by inappropriate conclusions, such as "There is no convincing evidence in the published literature to support the contention that exposures to ELF generated by sources such as household appliances (or) VDTs . . . are demonstrable health hazards."

➤ Lack of appropriate instruments and measurement guidelines, and a lack of communication with European laboratories that have the necessary technology and data.

➤ Not infrequent cognitive slippage that appears in the form of clunker assertions such as *EMF from VDTs cannot be harmful*

*because there are common household appliances that give
off more of it, or the chicken embryo and rat studies (which
showed EMF effects) are not relevant to human safety
concerns* (paraphrased from Oak Ridge, COT, and IBM sources).

Contorted reasonings like these could be the product of
motives more honorable than simple cover-up as suggested by
Brodeur. They could be the product of a diplomatic agenda of
compromise, of a reluctance to displease or frighten others
with scary news, or perhaps honest self-delusion.

➤ The cacophony of many voices, or many mirrors. Rommel had
some success during the desert wars in fooling his opponent
into thinking his tank forces were very numerous and on all
sides, by having trucks churn clouds of dust all around.
Comparable to that strategy, we have what appears to be
several legions of prominent institutions actively issuing
authoritative statements, providing testimony at legislative
hearings, publishing newsletters, and issuing press releases.
They have varied names: National Association of Manufacturers
(NAM), Electromagnetic Energy Policy Alliance (EEPA), Center
for Office Technology (COT), Computer and Business
Equipment Manufacturers Association (CBEMA), and so on ad
nauseam. But they have a common message of minimizing the
hazards of VDUs and blocking regulation. Since there is so
much agreement, they must be right. When you look inside the
front page of their newsletters you find a common list of
equipment manufacturing sponsors. Old Blue, for one, does a
lot of sponsoring, and they also allow their employees to serve
on committees that formulate standards. That is very generous.
ANSI/HFS 100 (1988) benefited from this assistance.

You have to admire the inside-outside strategy of the business
equipment manufacturers. So far it has worked. The prospect of a
general public fear and rejection of VDUs because of radiation has
been blunted and checkmated. While justifiable alarm over VDU EMF
is being controlled, the new units are being manufactured in
conformance with MPR II Limits—at least, all the new ones recently
checked by me. Before we know it we'll have little to worry about
from VDU radiation.

The Swedish strategy of public acknowledgment of the problem, and quick action to deal with it—also known as the "Tylenol strategy"—worked, but it was a lot less intriguing. It probably didn't cost much either. Just one problem, you guys: How many schools have those old monitors?

There may be an occasional skin rash, rhinitis, or other allergic condition that a worker suspects may be due to the VDU. Check the unit for EMF, and make sure it gets a thorough vacuuming every couple of months. VDUs attract and hold a lot of charged dust particles that can irritate allergies.

Part 2

Working conditions

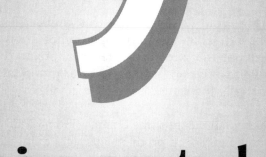

9

Noise control & privacy

CHAPTER 9

EVERY survey of office work conditions this writer has seen has listed distraction by noise as the number one source of work disruption and dissatisfaction (e.g., Brill 1984; Harris 1978).

The most oft-mentioned interrupters are people talking nearby, people talking on the phone, ringing phones (especially your own phone), and the noises from ventilation and office machines (copiers, printers, shredders). This does not particularly surprise the reader, because he or she knows from personal experience how disruptive extraneous conversations and ringing phones can be. In fact, entire mornings or afternoons, and sometimes even entire days, go by in which interruptions by people and telephones prevent getting anything started or finished. And you may frequently have to shut the door (if you are lucky enough to have one), find a quiet room, or go home to find the quiet and privacy needed to finish a project on time.

So you know this; your workers know this; and yet they must continue working in what are noisy, open office areas with five- to eight-foot partitions that provide some visual privacy but no noise protection or voice privacy. Even when your group moves, the new digs will be basically the same, just a little smaller.

What will it take to stimulate some change? Some hard data showing how noisy conditions reduce productivity might help, along with some numbers. But still the directive suggesting changes will have to come from above, as from the CEO or a VP. Well, at least we can provide some pretty hard data. DeMarco and Lister (1987) report on a survey of programmer productivity they have been conducting. Six hundred programmers from ninety-two companies were involved in timed tasks of programming speed and accuracy. They found a 10-to-1 difference between the best and worst programmers. They found that the worst programmers worked in noisy conditions where they were frequently interrupted. The companies with the quietest, least interruptive working conditions produced the most productive programmers. The average productivity of the top 25 percent was 2.6 times (260 percent) better than the bottom 25 percent. The two quartiles differed significantly on privacy and quietness measurements such as the following:

➤ Is your workspace acceptably quiet?

➤ Is your workspace acceptably private?

➤ Can you silence your phone?

➤ Can you forward your calls?

➤ Do people often interrupt you needlessly?

➤ How much dedicated work space do you have?

The top quartile averaged 78 square feet of space; the bottom quartile averaged 46 square feet.

On average, a knowledge worker (engineer, programmer, graphic designer, ergonomist) will be paid about $20 (including benefits) for every dollar spent on his or her workspace. A reasonable difference in productivity between a noisy, cramped workspace and a quieter one, with 25 to 30 square feet of work surface, is 300 percent. By reducing the size of a workspace and removing privacy walls you might be able to save a dollar on workspace and lose only seven dollars in productivity.

You really need to start with a survey and meetings with your workers. Find out what the interrupters and distracters are and start fixing them. Some of the important ones may not be expensive at all. For example, install call-forwarding and e-mail.

The office printers, copiers, shredders, and doors may be serious distracters for those who are located nearby. Many can be moved out of the work area, perhaps around the corner into the congregation area where the mail room and coffee pot are located. Or, the machines can be collected and walled in.

You should try to provide those who want it with thirty square feet of work surface. Sometimes this can be achieved by having workers put their archive files in a common filing area. Rolling files are a very space-economical way to store project files that may be needed later, or reference materials that are used only once in a while.[1]

If sound-deadening walls (floor-to-ceiling, preferably) absolutely cannot be provided for those workers needing them, then perhaps

1 E.G. Spacesaver Corp., 1450 Janesville Ave., Fort Atkinson, WI 53538-2798, 414-563-6363.

several quiet privacy offices can be shared. Workers needing privacy and quiet to finish a project on time can sign up to use one for a couple of days. They could also be used for meetings with customers in private. Priority and scheduling problems are predictable, but solvable.

Academic research has refined our knowledge of the manner in which noise, especially meaningful spoken conversation, distracts (Smith 1989). It disrupts encoding (information input) and decoding (output formulation). In other words, it interrupts learning, comprehending, and organizing your thoughts for reproduction. That's nice to know, but another finding has an important application. Geen (1984) showed that the temperament dimension of introversion-extroversion is important to consider in predicting response to potentially distracting noise. Introverts (quiet, self-sufficient) work better in quiet and are more disrupted by noise than extroverts. Extroverts prefer noisy interaction with others, work better with higher noise levels, and often find quiet conditions quite disturbing. The application comes when you decide where to locate work areas for certain individuals. I'm a frequent witness to Alex Extrovert's carrying on loud conversations with others while sitting just eight feet from Andy Introvert, who is trying to complete some kind of complicated fault-tree analysis. Andy has taken to wearing large ear muffs like those you see on the airport tarmac. The others worry too much about looking silly with those things on their head. In situations like this, a floor-to-ceiling wall between such obvious introverts and extroverts might not be a bad idea.

Providing floor-to-ceiling walls, and a door, is not an expensive proposition. Plasterboard makes an excellent sound-deadening wall (Fig. 9-1). You can get enough plasterboard (160 square feet) for an 80 square-foot office for less than $200 (in Minneapolis, anyway). If you want more flexibility in moving walls, you can get movable full-length walls from Clestra-Hauserman.[2]

Plan for some ventilation and overhead lighting in these offices. Without supplementary ventilation, putting up floor-to-ceiling walls

2 Clestra Hauserman Inc., 29525 Fountain Parkway, Solon, OH 44139-4351, 216-498-5088.

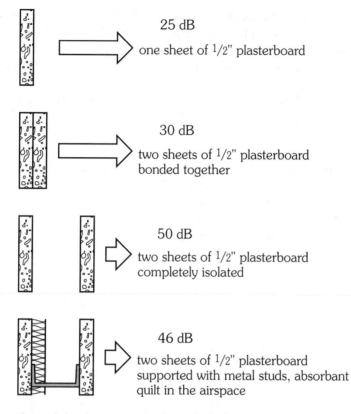

Figure 9-1

25 dB
one sheet of 1/2" plasterboard

30 dB
two sheets of 1/2" plasterboard
bonded together

50 dB
two sheets of 1/2" plasterboard
completely isolated

46 dB
two sheets of 1/2" plasterboard
supported with metal studs, absorbant
quilt in the airspace

Sound-deadening with plasterboard.

can create a stuffy work area. You might want to try noise-masking
first, before going to walls.

Background sound is a common method of masking the disturbing
noise in open plan areas. White noise is a better masker than
background music. Technical experts in the field of sound control[3]
should be consulted for this. They have the necessary instruments for
installing and adjusting the system. A good masking system can
significantly expand the "non-distraction buffer" around a worker. For
example, instead of being distracted by a conversation 14 ft. away,
the worker would not be distracted until the conversation moved
within 12 feet.

3 For example, Orfield Associates, Inc., 2709 E. 25th St., Minneapolis, MN 55406.

Additional inexpensive measures can help lower distracting noise. You can put up signs, with big shhh pictograms on them, and you can assist workers in arranging their workspace so that they face away from each other and are located the maximum distance from each other. This may provide a bit of telephone privacy, at least. The daily telephone soaps from neighboring cubicles can get a bit ragged. (On the other hand, the other guy's calling card number could come in handy!)

The reader may note the absence of any mention of standards for general office noise level. If you must have one, use the West German standard of 55 dB. However, the best standard to use is the one that satisfies the needs of your employees for productive work. Talk to them and find out what distracts them.

10

Lighting & windows

MOST office work areas are too brightly lit for work with VDUs. The overhead fluorescent lighting has not been designed, by way of intensity or position, for computer work. Sunlight from windows often presents problems with viewing the VDU screen. The more common problems and a common solution are presented below.

Figure 10-1 shows a generally diffuse, washed-out appearance of the VDU screen. An operator will have to get pretty close to the screen in order to read the text being displayed. The diffuse illumination comes from a generally high level of illumination in the work area, reflecting off the display.

Figure 10-1

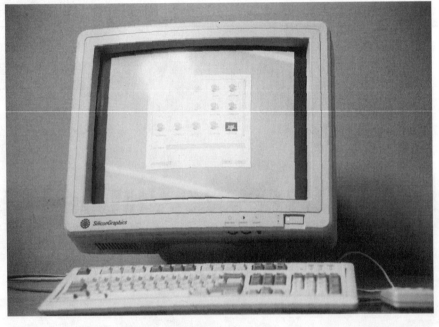

Washed-out display: diffuse reflected glare.

If you look closely at the upper left corner of the display you will see a big fuzzy blob of light coming from one of the overhead light fixtures. If we turn the display off you can see the fuzzy, reflected image of the fixture more clearly in Fig. 10-2.

Figure 10-2

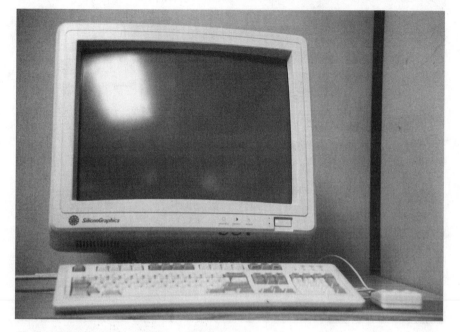

Reflected glare: out of focus light fixture.

Fixtures are seen more clearly in Fig. 10-3 where they are the subject of focus. An operator's eyes tend to focus on such reflected images, making the displayed text harder to read.

A third kind of glare problem is illustrated in Fig. 10-4. This is the direct glare of a light source shining into the operator's eyes.

An operator working under these conditions will experience a great deal of eyestrain because the eye muscles that control pupil size must constantly work to reduce the amount of light entering the eye. Also, squinting is hard work. The struggle to perceive text and images through the haze of glare reduces blinking, and produces dry, itchy eyes. Consequently, you will observe these poor souls frequently looking away from the screen and rubbing their eyes.

Quite often sore neck, shoulder, and arm muscles, and ulnar-compression symptoms, can be traced to lighting problems. The subject of Fig. 3-2 (page 41), shown propping herself up by her

Figure 10-3

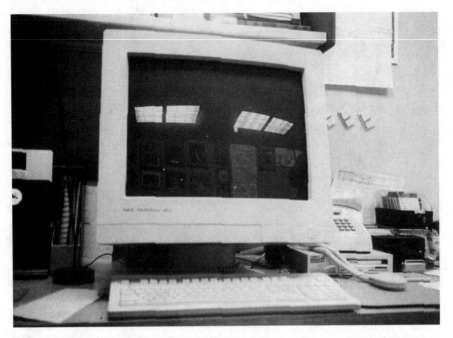

Reflected glare: focus on fixtures.

Figure 10-4

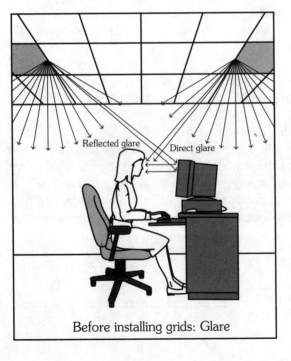

Before installing grids: Glare

Direct and reflected glare, before installing parasquare grid.

elbows, was using that posture to get her eyes close enough to read text on a washed-out display. Solving her lighting problem helped her neck and arm pains.

An adequate solution to glare problems has been achieved by turning off some of the fixtures, or disconnecting some of the tubes, to reduce the general light level, and then using Parasquare grids to redirect the light from other fixtures. Parasquare grids are honeycomb-looking arrays of small squares (or hexagons) that prevent light from the fixture spreading out at an angle of more than 30° to 45°. Deeper squares will restrict the angle more than shallow squares. Figure 10-5 shows how you receive light from the fixture if you are close to it. When you move just a few feet away (Fig. 10-6) the light is blocked from view, and from shining into your screen or eyes if you are working at your VDT.

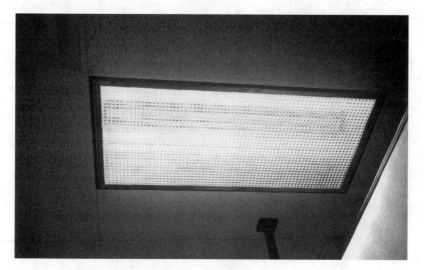

Figure 10-5

Light coming through parasquare grid.

I've been able to solve most glare problems by reducing the level of overhead illumination, turning off some fixtures or tubes, and by putting Parasquare grids on fixtures that were creating direct or reflected-glare problems for the operator. These solutions are illustrated in Figs. 10-6, 10-7, 10-8, and 10-9. If you have the rare opportunity to investigate new lighting concepts, look at polarized

Figure 10-6

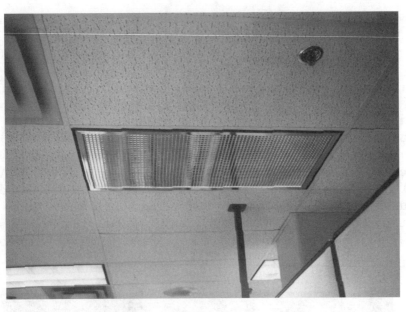

Light blocked by parasquare grid.

Figure 10-7

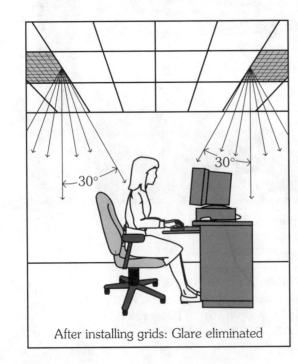

Direct and reflected glare, glare eliminated after installing parasquare grid.

After installing grids: Glare eliminated

Figure 10-8

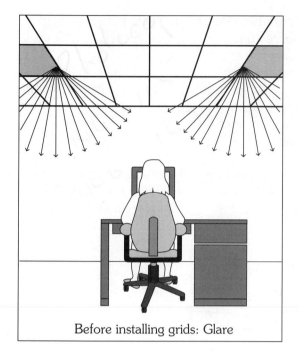

Before installing grids: Glare

Reflected and ambient glare from the side, before installing parasquare grid.

Figure 10-9

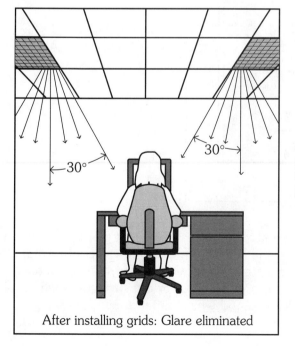

After installing grids: Glare eliminated

Reflected and ambient glare from the side, eliminated after installing parasquare grid.

lighting or a lens system (lensed indirect lighting) that spreads light upward and evenly over the ceiling.

If eliminating the glare problems for a given worker has required reducing ambient light below a level that provides comfortable reading of paper documents, then task lighting in the form of desk lamps can be used where needed. Some workers prefer incandescent over fluorescent lamps for this purpose.

Task lighting supplied as part of some panel systems does not work well, because too much light is then directed toward the worker (Fig. 10-10). The light should be directed away from the reader.

Figure 10-10

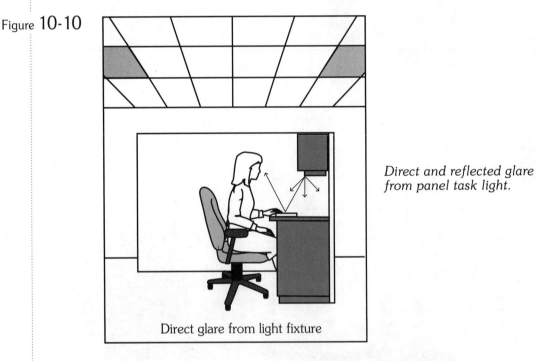

Direct and reflected glare from panel task light.

Direct glare from light fixture

The VDU itself can be a source of unnecessary direct glare. Sometimes operators forget that they have a brightness control that can be used to reduce direct screen glare. Other controllable sources of glare include reflections from polished or bright surfaces, such as ceilings, floors, walls, desk tops, and white paper documents.

Matte surfaces reduce reflected glare. Dark surfaces reduce glare; however, an old human factors saw says that a lot of contrast between light surfaces (VDU, paper, lamps) and dark surfaces (desk, table, cubicle walls) in the working visual field is not recommended because it causes a lot of strain on the pupils as the eye moves from light to dark surfaces. This may be true, but it may be more of a strain working with surfaces that are all too bright and require constant contractions of the pupils. Research by Haubner and Kokoschka (1983), reported by Grandjean (1987, p. 44), suggests that a mix of light and dark surfaces does not produce subjective eye discomfort. So, let the individual worker's preference be your guide on this point as well as others. The important point is that the worker should be able to relax back, beyond 90° in his chair, and comfortably view text on the screen without squinting, straining, or leaning toward the screen. Also, make sure none of your employees sees flickering of the fluorescent lights. This can be a source of eyestrain even for those who don't consciously see it. Their eyes still react to it.

Sunlight can be a significant source of glare (all types), for those lucky enough to have windows. Figure 10-11 shows some of the

Figure 10-11

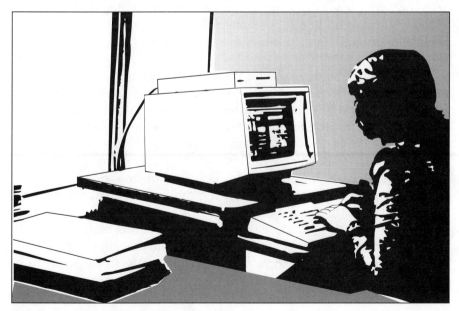

Direct and reflected glare from windows.

consequences of poor VDU placement vis-a-vis windows. The windows are producing direct glare, causing the operator to hunch over the keyboard and put her face close to the screen in order to read the video text. She will develop neck, shoulder, and back pain if she keeps her VDU near the window. If she puts her VDU against one of the other three walls, the window light will provide a source of reflected glare off the screen and bright walls.

So, how do you deal with bright sunlight? There are solutions, such as drawing the curtains. But that is an unhappy solution because it eliminates the treasure of sunlight and a view. Happier solutions may involve putting light-control film or polarizing film on the windows. This reduces the brightness but retains the view. You can get these at a photography supply store. Or, vertical blinds can be drawn so that sunlight is directed away from the VDU, toward back walls.

If you have a choice of installing vertical or horizontal blinds in your windows, select vertical ones. They are more effective in directing sunlight away from your screen without requiring you to shut the blinds entirely.

An important benefit of a sunlit room is the cost saving that comes from not turning on lights. A smallish 2 × 4-foot window provides more than enough light for an average-to-large office.

Glare shields and screens put on the VDU reduce image sharpness somewhat, and are recommended only when other methods of reducing glare are not adequate. Workers with windows often prefer a glare shield to drawing the blinds. If you are looking at glare shields and screens, forget about the mesh screen variety. They reduce image sharpness more than coated shields and they collect dust in a hurry. Look at a variety of different shields before choosing. Some coatings are greasy and hold fingerprints forever, and some retain more image sharpness than others.

I saw one shield advertised as clarifying (i.e., increasing image sharpness) and sent away for it.[1] The clarifying effect has yet to appear after a week of use, but it does seem to produce minimal

1 Less Gauss, Inc., P. O. Box 5006, Rhinebeck, NY 12572, 800-872-2005.

image degradation. Look for the American Optometric Association (AOA) seal of acceptance on a shield. Their approval means the shield is effective. Grandjean (1987, p. 85) suggests that a circular polarizing filter with an anti-reflection coating may do the best job of retaining image sharpness, but they do tend to be expensive.

Some glare screens are advertised as screening out harmful radiation as well as glare. They don't help. If you look closely at the advertising statements, you will see that the radiation blocked is electrical radiation, which is not suspected of having harmful biological effects. The suspected harmful radiation is magnetic radiation, which is not screened out (Pearce 1992). You can protect yourself adequately from magnetic radiation by staying at least 24 inches from the front of the monitor and 40 inches from its sides and back.

Dust and demagnetize (deGauss) your monitor every day. Check to see if you have a deGauss button on the back of your monitor. Some models deGauss automatically when turned on.

If all of these measures fail to provide a satisfactory image, you may need a better monitor.

⇨ Selecting a VDU to minimize glare & eyestrain

Video text takes longer to read than printed text. The characters tend to be a bit fuzzier than the printed word, and levels of contrast and brightness can be out of adjustment. This makes VDUs harder on the eyes than reading the printed word. One big difference lies in how you improve focus. With the printed word you move it toward or away from your eyes. With current computer designs you have to bend your body over the keyboard to bring the text into good focus. So, these disadvantages of the VDU are obvious, but they are not causing people to throw out their VDUs. The advantages of computers are too numerous to allow that. The visual quality of the newer VDUs is improving, and the larger screen sizes can help provide larger characters for more comfortable viewing.

It is now generally recognized that prolonged computer use during the day leads to eyestrain, blurred vision, burning eyes, light sensitivity, trouble with depth perception, double images, and other vision problems.[2,3] The basic reason for this lies in the design of the human eye. Until the newborn infant is about one month old, objects about 19 centimeters away are in focus. For the fully developed human eye, with the eye relaxed, objects in the distance are in focus. This is called the resting point of accommodation. To focus on near objects, ciliary muscles surrounding the iris of the eye contract to change the shape of the lens from flat to more nearly round. Other eye muscles constantly at work are the iris muscles that open and close the pupil in response to changing light levels, and oculometer muscles that move the eyeball up and down, and side to side, as you track images on the screen or look from screen to copy.

Thus, when you are viewing a computer screen or are looking at material in a copy holder, the ciliary and other eye muscles are in a constant state of tension. With bright lighting and screen glare, the effort required to bring objects into focus increases. Eye fatigue becomes significant within fifteen minutes. No wonder eyestrain, headache, and blurred vision are the most frequent complaints of computer users. The American Optometric Association recommends taking a 15-minute alternate task break every hour. They also recommend an ambient light level of 20 to 50 foot candles (which is about half the level used in most offices) for a computer workstation.[4]

Since close computer work puts so much strain on eye muscles, and eye-muscle fatigue is a general condition of computer work, employees must obtain thorough eye exams and have treatment or corrections for nearsightedness, farsightedness, astigmatism, amblyopia (lack of eye coordination), hyperopia (each eye sees things at a different level, causing head tilting), and other vision problems.

2 *VDT User's Guide to Better Vision*, 1992, American Optometric Association, St. Louis, MO 63141, 314-991-4100.

3 J. A. Sheedy, "Vision Problems at Video Display Terminals: A Survey of Optometrists," *Journal of the American Optometric Association*, 1992, Vol. 63: 687–92.

4 A simple test to see if you need to lower the light level in your workstation. Shade your eyes with your hands. If you feel your eyes relax your lights are too bright.

Otherwise, these defects will multiply the strain and fatigue of VDU work.

Most computer work does not require a color monitor. The use of color adds another source of eyestrain, since some colors (e.g., blues) tend to focus in front of the retina and others (reds) tend to focus in back of the retina. Thus, using blue images causes ciliary muscles to work extra hard to bulge the lens out to focus the images on the retina. Also, color monitors are more expensive to purchase and operate. The most eye-comfortable colors are black characters on gray background, followed by gray on white, yellow on green, and light green on dark green.

Special glasses are often prescribed for computer users to help relieve some of the visual and postural strains. There are a variety of prescription types; for example, single-correction computer lenses are sometimes prescribed for bifocal wearers. Sometimes special bifocals are also prescribed for bifocal wearers. Because the VDU, copyholder, and keyboard are farther away than typical reading material the correction for near vision in computer bifocals should be different than for street bifocals.

Other types of computer glasses are available. For example, progressive addition lenses (PALs) provide a smooth correction from top to bottom as the gaze is lowered from distant to near objects. A computer-specific PAL would provide correction for the VDU with a slight depression of gaze. Additional gaze lowering would provide gaze correction for the keyboard and desktop.

There does seem to be limits, however, to the use of glasses in solving VDU problem. The trouble with the current approach to computer glasses is that they are made for viewing screen and keyboard each from a specific distance. This tends to increase rigidity and inactivity while working. Given the importance of a leaning-back posture, and of varying the back angle during the day, computer glasses should have a correction for viewing the screen from a leaning-back posture as well as a more upright angle.

A frequent computer user, and a manager of computer users, should seek out more detail on computers and visual stress. Readable discussions of vision problems and computer glasses have appeared in the journal, *Occupational Health and Safety.*[5,6] A recent paperback book by an optometrist (Goding and Hacunda 1993) provides more detail, additional references, and some exercises for strengthening eye muscles.

Computer models will differ in these characteristics:

➢ Screen brightness. The screen should not flicker or fluctuate. The monitor should have a screen refresh rate of 65 cycles per second or higher to prevent flicker.

➢ Edge sharpness of characters, which affects the crispness of character definition. Dot matrix size should be at least 7×9.

➢ Image contrast, which refers to the brightness difference between image and background—dark black characters against a white background, for example, as opposed to dark gray against light gray. There should be control knobs for brightness and contrast adjustments.

➢ Screen size and character size. Character-size criteria specified by the New York City schools (4.1 millimeter) and LOHP[7] (3/16 inch) are very close to each other, and are good criteria for minimum character size. You can enlarge characters with some operating systems, such as the Mac System 7 or Microsoft Windows. A multiresolution monitor will permit enlarging characters by enlarging the pixels.

➢ Image stability. Characters can seem to move (drift or jitter) or be out of alignment on a poor monitor.

➢ Spacing between characters, words, and lines of text. Too little space can create visual strain.

➢ Flat screens create less character distortion than curved ones.

➢ Availability of many character fonts. Having several to choose from can be helpful.

5 R. Van Stroh, "Computer Vision Syndrome," *Occupational Health and Safety*, October 1993, 62–66.

6 L. K. Wan, "Task-Specific Glasses: Understanding Needs, Reaping Benefits," *Occupational Health and Safety*, March 1992, 50–52.

7 The Labor Occupational Health Program at the University of California, Berkeley, CA 94720, 415-642-5507.

> ➤ Meet Swedish MPR II, or TCO, guidelines for radiation-emission limits.

> ➤ Compare a prospective new monitor against your best old one and against other new ones. It should have better character definition and readability than the others. Salesmen don't always show their best quality monitors first.

> ➤ Check computer magazines such as *PC Week* or *Mac World* for annual reviews of monitor quality. Sony seems to rank high consistently on these reviews. For more detail on monitor qualities consult ANSI/HFS 100 (1988) or Snyder, 1986.

⇨ Windows

People like windows and sunlight. After working all day in an almost windowless environment, how cheering it is to walk out into a sunny world, even in the winter. You know this and your workers know this. The whole world knows this; at least we can be sure the Danes do, since by law they do not permit windowless workrooms.

There are a few problems with windows, such as temperature and light control. When asked why they like windows, people talk about sunlight and the view of an interesting world. The workers most unhappy about the lack of windows are those with repetitive, monotonous jobs (Collins 1975).

Some evidence even exists that a window view can help restore health. Roger Ulrich (1989) examined hospital records for gall bladder patients in a suburban Pennsylvania hospital. He compared records of those who had rooms with an outside view of trees against those who had an outside view of a brick wall. Those with the view of trees had shorter hospital stays, required less pain medication, and made fewer criticisms of the nurses.

The BOSTI study (Brill 1984) found that most office workers (60 percent) could see a window from their workspace. Nearly half (47 percent) were within ten feet of one. How does your area compare to that?

These are the main reasons for having a window nearby:

➢ Close work, such as reading or using a VDU, puts strain on the eye muscles of accommodation required for near focus. Opthamologists (e.g., Sussman and Loewenstein 1993) and optometrists recommend turning away from close work and looking into the distance, such as out a window, every two to three minutes. To prevent fatigue of eye muscles they also recommended certain eye exercises.

➢ A lot of office work is boring, and windows provide boredom relief. Even interesting work can become boring after a while, simply because of the sameness of the work. A refreshing look out of a window (not at a brick wall) for a few minutes can re-establish an interest in what you are doing.

➢ Your workers want it. Almost universally. There is probably more to this than we understand right now.

Temperature

Quite a bit of evidence has now established what we know from common experience: that being too hot causes sleepiness, increased errors, and reduced performance. On the other hand, being too cold induces restlessness, distraction, and thus reduces performance on mental tasks. However, you may find the following experiment interesting. Find the temperature at which workers have no sense of temperature at which they are very thermally comfortable. Now turn the thermostat down one degree Fahrenheit. They should be a bit more productive, yet there will be few if any complaints about temperature. And there should be less napping.

If any of your workers feel cold, turn the temperature up. Working in cold temperatures increases the likelihood of carpal tunnel syndrome and other CTDs.

Computer diddling? Not here!

An accounting software company in Sausalito, California, SBT Corp., estimates that business computers are involved in nonwork-related activity an average of 5.1 hours per week.[8] They estimated that "PC futzing" like this costs U.S. business $100 billion per year, which is two percent of the gross domestic product. However, that becomes a pretty empty figure when you look at what they mean by futzing. They define it as waiting for programs to run or documents to be printed, waiting on hold for help with a problem, checking and formatting documents, loading and learning new programs, helping co-workers with problems, organizing and erasing files, and only 17 percent in playing games.

Futzing is what has to be done to get computers to work. It's no more wasted time than is keeping your car in good repair. This confirms the line on bean counters—that you don't let them stray too far from their numbers. They can be dangerous if you let them make business decisions. The 17 percent is what we call diddling, not futzing.

What's wrong with having a little fun with your computer? There's that neat game of solitaire that came with Microsoft Windows that Ray has been working on. Microsoft said it is educational and will help users learn how to use a mouse. It's been about a year since Ray got it. He practices every day. I'll bet he's a pretty good mouse user now. Another popular Microsoft game is minesweeper, in which one tries to uncover land mines without being blown up.

People are meeting and courting on the Internet these days. They said to get a life, didn't they? They're breaking up, too. Jo-Anne found out that her Internet steady was e-mailing other girls, and broke it off.

Even the reader probably does a bit of diddling. Anyone who'd pick up a book with "PC" in the title probably diddles. But if this is a problem at your workplace, I have a solution. It's a privacy filter made by 3M![9] People who walk by your cubicle or office won't be able to see what you're doing (Fig. 10-12).

8 Reported by J. Panettier, *Information Week*, September 6, 1993, pp. 33–37.

9 3M Safety and Security Division, 3M Center, Bldg. 225-4N-14, St. Paul, MN 55144-1000, 800-553-9215.

Figure 10-12

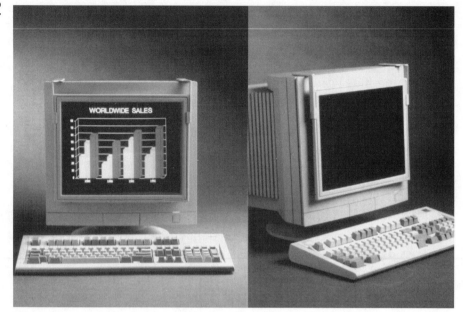

3M privacy filter.

11

Productivity gains from using groupware

I F you work with others, groupware is one of the best possible tools for boosting your productivity.

⇨ What is groupware?

Groupware lets network users share information with each other and monitor workflow. Groupware includes:

➤ E-mail

➤ Basic groupware such as Lotus Notes

➤ Workflow software

➤ Personal information managers (PIMs)

➤ Meeting software

➤ Multimedia

➤ Group authoring software

Groupware gives workers a system for managing relationships with other workers. It also gives them consistent, current databases to use. Best of all, it lets them manage time and space without worrying about where other workers are, or even when they will be working.

Groupware allows rapid, informal organization of new workgroups. It makes the ubiquitous computer possible.

⇨ E-mail

E-mail is the most limited kind of groupware. Unlike other groupware, e-mail cannot route information from many persons to many other persons (many-to-many communication). However, it can route information from one person to another (one-to-one communication) or from one person to many others (one-to-many). Its mechanisms for attaching files to e-mail are primitive, too. The price is right, though. Anything more sophisticated requires software such as Lotus Notes, at the cost of a few hundred dollars per network node.

⇨ Basic groupware

Lotus Notes dominates the category of basic groupware. Lotus Development Corporation introduced it in 1989 (Taber 1992). By late 1993 it had sold more than 500,000 copies to more than 2500 companies (Kirkpatrick 1993).

Notes is for developing and using groupware applications. It offers full text-search capability, automatic versioning of documents, database replication, application development tools, administrative tools, backend services, and network support.

Notes combines a message system with a large database that contains work records and memos. It also provides a corporate on-line service that lets users read from (or write to) bulletin boards. It has a centralized data dictionary that lets users share files across multiple LANs. This gives Notes servers a directory of users and files.

Notes monitors e-mail and work-in-progress. It also handles correspondence and maintains informal databases. It provides users a way to store documents that have relationships to each other.

Notes is useful for tracking events, broadcasting information, supporting on-going discussions, and providing reference material to widely dispersed users.

Notes users can follow business activities such as sales or purchases. They can make announcements or post information to databases. Notes users can also sift through information such as sales reports. They can discuss business in either an ad hoc or a structured manner.

Notes is primarily for applications that rely on text, not numbers. It is strongest at broadcasting information, especially for laptop users who need access to the same information that is available to desktop computer users. Notes' full text-search capability lets users do fully integrated text indexing and searching. This speeds database queries.

Applications that require on-line transaction processing (OLTP), in which databases are updated for each transaction, are unsuited for Notes because Notes databases are updated only at intervals.

Notes supports AppleTalk, Netware, TCP\IP, X.25, SNA, Pathworks, NetBIOS, and VINES. Administrative tools available with Notes include remote management capability. A hierarchical naming scheme makes Notes easier for administrators to manage.

Notes programmers can choose a subset of documents to replicate, or they can replicate an entire database. Notes can do these replications in either the foreground or the background.

Among the tools for building Notes applications are Notes APIs. There are Notes APIs for project tracking, forms routing, and custom buttons for options based on formulas and for forms authorization. There is built-in Vendor Independent Messaging (VIM) mail support. This can be used for routing forms from place to place.

Personal information managers (PIMs)

Shared contact information and group scheduling are the heart of networked (i.e., workgroup) PIMs. This software offers important advantages over paper-based systems. It is easier to use, quicker, and more accurate.

PIM buyers should look for:

> ➤ Remote access capability
> ➤ Communication between laptop and desktop computers
> ➤ Context-sensitive help
> ➤ Image-data-handling capability
> ➤ Multiple databases
> ➤ Concurrent use of databases
> ➤ Ability to customize views of data
> ➤ Group scheduling

➤ Communication with other applications

➤ Data import/export capability

➤ Gantt charting capability

➤ User-customizable templates for contact management, logging telephone calls, and scheduling

➤ Automatic triggering of such events as auto-dialing or sending e-mail

Networked PIMs can create logs for managers to use to keep track of work processes. Networked PIMs can create logs of telephone calls and calendar changes that show day-to-day activity.

The best reason, though, for buying networked PIMs is data security. Salespeople who leave a company can take all their client contact information with them if their PIMs are not networked, but not if they have been using networked PIMs. Also, in the latter case, new salespeople can take up right where their predecessors leave off.

⇨ Workflow software

Workflow software divides worker's interactions with other workers into manageable steps. This helps workers understand the steps needed to get jobs done. Workflow software maps the interactions between workers. This helps them discover problem areas and record solutions to these problems for future reference.

Workflow software eliminates unnecessary steps. It also ensures that all necessary steps are executed. It improves quality, reduces errors in communication, and shortens the time needed to complete projects. Workflow software streamlines and automates business processes. It also automatically routes forms from one worker to another. It can store and forward data from one member of a workgroup to another when a triggering event, such as completion of a form, occurs.

Workflow-analysis diagrams show the role of everyone involved in a work process. This makes it possible to keep track of each worker's contribution to a job.

✳ Desirable features for workflow software

Workflow software should:

➤ Promote ad hoc workflow

➤ Let managers set up project due dates

➤ Let managers make task assignments

➤ Show the life cycles of documents

➤ Support automatic message sending

➤ Create a history log for each project

➤ Answer project status queries

➤ Support dynamic forms that display different fields, depending on who is working on a form

➤ Permit the attachment of routing instructions to forms

➤ Allow definition of summary statistics

➤ Provide audit trails

➤ Provide a high-level scripting language to define forms

➤ Provide a high-level scripting language to define workflow

✳ A case study of workflow software

Before buying workflow software, determine if there is room for improvement. Workflow software can bring big benefits but it takes lots of work. For example, Chuck Riley, group director and vice president of Young & Rubicam advertising agency, worked with his staff and Action Technologies employees to analyze workflow at the ad agency. His team interviewed many workers to determine the workflow pattern at the agency. He learned that gaps in information often forced workers to backtrack after projects were underway. Once Riley's team knew about this problem it was able to design procedures to ensure that workers would always have the information they needed.

⇨ Meeting software

Meeting software lets participants in conferences or face-to-face meetings use personal computers to "talk" at the same time. Meetings that use meeting software go faster because users are able to read faster than they can talk and because they do not have to wait for others to finish talking before replying. Meeting software lets quiet, less-assertive people contribute to meetings. In this way it equalizes participation. Much conversation in an electronic meeting is anonymous. This makes rank less important.

Meeting software aids groups in generating new ideas, outlining alternatives, building workgroup consensus, choosing alternatives, making plans, and making accurate transcripts of meetings.

Meeting software frees users from attending lengthy meetings filled with agenda items that do not concern them. Users can participate in discussions at times that are most convenient. They can take phone calls during virtual meetings or do other work while monitoring discussions.

Meeting software is especially valuable for strategic planning, workgroup development, training, quality control, personnel evaluation, and compensation management. Meeting software is best for electronic meetings whose purpose is technical. Lack of information about body language (posture, facial expressions, and the like) makes this software less useful for meetings that involve emotion—negotiations, for example.

Taligent, Inc., the joint effort by Apple and IBM to create a new operating system, has benefited from using an electronic conferencing program. Taligent managers found that they could eliminate many meetings, yet provide an important way to foster communication between workers and management (LaPlante 1993). Taligent workers use a bulletin board to exchange a wide range of information. The bulletin board also gives management up-to-the-minute information about software development. It gives individual engineers a way to exchange information, too. Taligent management feel that their on-line bulletin board displays the pattern of interactions between workers, thereby showing the status of projects better than memos or reports would do. The bulletin board allows users to attach documents, drawings, and sound. It also provides an introduction to the company for new employees.

⇨ Multimedia

Multimedia can help transform networks of personal computers into distributed work environments that are ideal for collaborative projects. By combining images, text, sound, color animation, and full-motion video, multimedia can add value to:

➢ Audiovisual presentations

➢ Databases

➢ Desktop video conferencing

➢ Desktop video production

➢ Education and training

➢ Electronic newsletters

➢ E-mail

➢ Information services

➢ Groupware

➢ Teleconferencing and more

Mixing color animation, text, sound, and full-motion video can make complex ideas simple. It can make abstract information concrete. It can also make software applications easier to learn. By speeding learning it can increase productivity.

Using full-motion video comes at a price, though. One minute of full-motion video requires a large amount of storage space. This ranges from about 500 thousand bytes for low-quality video to 10 megabytes for VHS-quality video.

Apart from its use in education, multimedia will find one of its biggest uses in teleconferencing, where it will add behavioral cues whose richness approaches those available in face-to-face meetings.

In the future, teleconferencing participants will be able to share animation, data files, graphics, stored audio, and video. Participants will be able to annotate documents, including diagrams, charts and graphs, memos, and spreadsheets.

Major effects of groupware

Groupware has powerful effects. It flattens organization hierarchies, makes work more flexible, and frees workers from noise and other interruptions. It also makes telecommuting easier.

Flatter hierarchies

Groupware helps workers share knowledge, and knowledge is power. So groupware means power sharing. This flattens hierarchies in organizations.

Flexibility

Groupware makes it possible to assemble a workgroup fast and disband it fast when work is done.

Noise control

The only real excuse for using open office layouts has been the need to rearrange work spaces when old workgroups are disbanded and new workgroups are created. Short, flimsy partitions are easier to move than solid walls that go all the way to the ceiling, so this reasoning goes. With groupware substituting for many face-to-face meetings, the problems of controlling noise and distraction can be resolved by moving workers to private offices that have solid walls and doors that close.

⇨ Increased support for telecommuting

Groupware can keep track of each worker's contribution to a project. Since groupware can track individual workers it tells managers about talented workers whom they otherwise might never know. Groupware also lets managers know what workers are doing, out in the field. This makes them more willing to let workers telecommute.

Groupware fuels explosive growth in telecommuting. Four million American workers were telecommuting by the end of 1990, a year after Lotus introduced Notes. This number rose above 8.3 million by the beginning of 1994 (Kotkin 1994), a growth rate of more than 44 percent a year.

⇨ Productivity gains from telecommuting

Telecommuting is bringing big gains in worker productivity. For example, the Los Angeles County Assessor's office found that telecommuters process their work 64 percent faster than office-bound workers (Kotkin 1994). The overall productivity of the Assessor's office rose by 34 percent after its workers began telecommuting.

American Express had similar productivity gains in a test project at one of its facilities (Sherman 1993). It found that travel reservation agents who work from home handle 26 percent more calls at home than they do at the office. This has yielded a 46-percent increase in revenue per home worker.

American Express travel agent, Faye Compton, who works at home most days, says that her increased productivity results from the lack of distraction and a correspondingly enhanced ability to concentrate (Sherman 1993). Besides avoiding distractions by working at home she also avoids the fatigue, danger, and expense caused by commuting to the office.

⇨ Cost-cutting from increased telecommuting

American Express says that it expects its annual office rental cost savings to be $4400 per telecommuting worker in New York City. Jack Nilles, the Los Angeles consultant who is credited with first use of the term "telecommuting," says that companies can cut costs by $8000 a year for each mid-level employee who telecommutes regularly (Kotkin 1994).

⇨ Some productivity history

Dramatic productivity gains from using groupware contrast with what has been uniformly low white-collar productivity until recently. Writing in *The Economist* in 1990, Stephen Roach reported that the average output produced by white-collar workers was no greater in 1990 than it was in 1960. Roach noted that this is true even though office equipment comprised an 18-percent share of America's stock of fixed capital in 1990 (excluding real estate), a big increase from its 3-percent share in 1960. He calculated that by 1986 the average output of white-collar workers had fallen nearly 7 percent below the average output of white-collar workers in the 1970s, before the introduction of personal computers.

This steady, almost unchanging level of productivity contrasts sharply with the steadily rising productivity of computer programmers, with each new improvement in computers (see Chapter 12 for more details about programmer productivity). Probably, personal computers have been too complicated for the average white-collar worker to use, until recently, when graphic user interfaces replaced command-line user interfaces.

⇨ Productivity gains from using graphic interfaces

The Gartner Group, a consulting firm in Stamford, Connecticut, compared (Kirkpatrick 1993a) the five-year costs of owning and using

169

IBM-style PCs equipped with MS-DOS, IBM-style PCs equipped with Windows, and Macintosh computers equipped with Apple's graphically oriented operating system.

After counting all costs of personal computer use, including purchase price and costs of operation (administration, maintenance, supplies and training) the Gartner Group found that the total five-year cost was $25,000 per Macintosh user, $29,500 per Windows user, and $40,000 per MS-DOS user. Administrative, support and training costs accounted for these differences in total costs.

Management Today reports an interesting indication of the greater ease of use of a graphic user interface such as Windows or the Mac's interface, compared with using MS-DOS (Bird 1993). Windows users have an average of four applications installed. MS-DOS users have only 2.5 applications installed, on the average. It is as if an average of 2.5 MS-DOS applications is as many as computer workers can readily learn to use.

⇨ Productivity gains from using groupware

Although the switch from MS-DOS software to Windows-based software has produced dramatic gains, it is clear that groupware itself yields additional big gains. *Fortune* magazine reported Boeing experiments that measured productivity gains from using groupware (Kirkpatrick 1993b). According to *Fortune*, Boeing found it could shorten the development times for some projects by as much as 90 percent by using groupware.

This result agrees closely with the experience of the Marriott hotel chain. Carl DiPietro, manager of an electronic decision center for the chain, found that groupware let users complete meetings in one-tenth of the time they would normally have taken (Hamilton 1992).

⇨ A manager's checklist for making groupware work for you

These are the steps you need to take to make groupware work for your company:

> ➤ Establish specific goals
>
> ➤ Install the necessary groupware technology
>
> ➤ Appoint workgroup members
>
> ➤ Appoint workgroup editors
>
> ➤ Examine existing work processes
>
> ➤ Develop a pilot project
>
> ➤ Measure results
>
> ➤ Reward workgroup members

⇨ Establish specific goals

When you introduce groupware, begin by establishing highly specific goals. Aim to solve a core business problem. Don't aim for vague goals like "improved communication," or "more participation in meetings." Aim for concrete goals, such as shortening product development time or getting higher sales for a product line.

⇨ Install groupware technology

Workgroups often spread beyond a particular location. Install enough local-area networks and wide-area networks to support each member of each workgroup. Be sure to choose fast server computers. Choose fast client computers, too.

⇨ Appoint workgroup members

Create workgroups whose purpose is to reach a specific goal. Include workers from several different disciplines. Cut across established boundaries, if necessary. Expect workgroup membership to shift as tasks change.

⇨ Appoint workgroup editors

Groupware databases can become clogged with data. Trivial information can obscure important information. Appoint editors to remove incorrect or unnecessary material from databases.

⇨ Examine existing work processes

Interview workers, business managers, and information system experts to identify potential trouble spots in work processes. Identify the trouble spots in the system that you are using now. Carefully describe patterns of workflow.

⇨ Develop a pilot project

Don't expect to solve all of your problems at once. Start with a small problem that you're sure you can solve. Branch out gradually.

⇨ Design a training plan

Hold workshops to explain your new groupware system. Demonstrate groupware to groups of users. Hold in-house application-development courses for developers. Teach users good manners for using on-line systems. Use groupware to train new workers. Get them started quickly by letting them explore historical databases that show how your company works.

⇨ Measure results

Develop a clear picture of the situation that existed before you introduced groupware. Use this information to establish a baseline. Measure your results against the baseline. Make measurements frequently. Match progress reports to specific project goals.

⇨ Reward workgroup members

Design systems that make everyone's responsibility clear. Using workgroup software means sharing information. So, reward your workers for sharing information.

12

The importance
of speed

CHAPTER 12

If it were done when 'tis done, then 'twere well it were done quickly."
Macbeth, Act 1, Scene 7

A LMOST everyone knows that fast computers are more fun to use than slow ones, but few people seem to know just how much they can boost their productivity by using fast computers. Today, after decades of big increases in computer speed and productivity, it is still possible to find writers who say that computer users don't need fast computers for most of the work they want to do (Husted 1994).

The effects of computer speed

In the past, every increase in computer speed has boosted the productivity of computer programmers. As long ago as the 1960s, computer programmers who used on-line time-sharing systems were able to write and debug twice as much code each year as programmers who used batch processing methods. This is true even though time-sharing systems were slow, compared with today's personal computers. (Managers of time-sharing systems often aimed for average computer system response times of as much as four seconds or more.)

In an early experiment, programmers who used batch processing methods to debug programs took three times as long as programmers who used time-sharing terminals (Sackman eat al. 1968). This early experiment inspired a lot of research, including some key studies by IBM about the economic value of rapid response time (IBM 1982).

Brady (1986) summed up the best of this research in several graphs. Figure 12-1, redrawn from one of these graphs, shows that the productivity of highly-skilled programmers increases almost fivefold when average computer system response time falls from 1.5 seconds to 0.3 seconds.

Figure 12-2 shows what happens to the productivity of average programmers when average computer system response time falls from 1.5 seconds to 0.3 seconds. As you can see, this decrease of only 1.2

Figure 12-1

Productivity

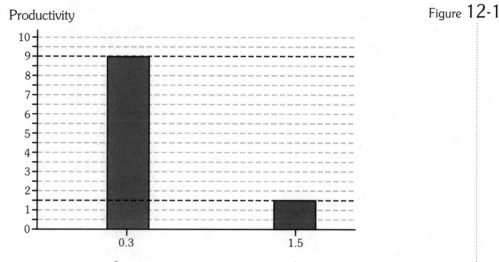

System response time, in seconds

Productivity of highly-skilled programmers.

Figure 12-2

Productivity

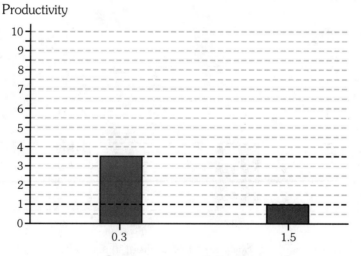

System response time, in seconds

Productivity of average programmers.

seconds gives average programmers roughly a three-fold increase in productivity. Evidently, you can increase productivity by supplying fast computers to those of your workers who have average skills. However, you can get much bigger gains by supplying these computers to your best workers instead (compare Fig. 12-1 and Fig. 12-2).

One way to see the extent of damage caused by long computer system response times is to adjust these response times to make the productivity of highly-skilled programmers equal to the productivity of average programmers (Fig. 12-3). Highly-skilled programmers who use computer systems that give an average response time of 0.7 seconds have the same productivity as average programmers whose computer systems give them an average response time of 0.3 seconds. Notice, too, that the productivity of highly-skilled programmers falls by two-thirds when average computer system response time increases from 0.3 seconds to 0.7 seconds (compare Fig. 12-1 and Fig. 12-3).

 Figure 12-3

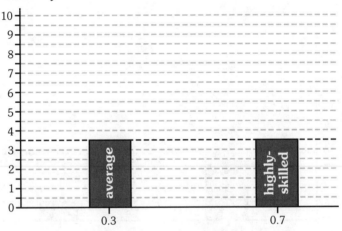

Productivity of average programmers and highly-skilled programmers.

The gap between the productivity of average programmers and highly-skilled programmers widens a great deal when computer speed increases. For example, if average system response time is 0.3 seconds, the productivity of highly-skilled programmers is almost three times greater than the productivity of average programmers. In contrast with this, the productivity of highly-skilled programmers is only about 50 percent greater than the productivity of average programmers when average computer system response times are 1.5 seconds (Fig. 12-1 and Fig. 12-2).

Other studies strongly indicate that computer delays reduce productivity. For example, Lambert (1984) found that programmer productivity, measured in lines of code written and debugged, increases by 58 percent when average computer system response time drops from 2.23 seconds to 0.84 seconds.

Most of the damage to productivity is done by average computer system response times that range from 0.3 seconds to about 0.7 seconds. Damage continues to increase, although more gradually, as computer system response time continues to increase past 0.7 seconds (Doherty and Keliskey 1979, Lambert 1984, Brady 1986, Thadhani 1981).

⇨ How to use research about computer speed

You can use research about computer speed and user-productivity to help you when you choose a computer expert. The secret is that few computer experts know about this research, because it is about human brains and not computers. Here is a list of articles about computer speed and user productivity that you can use to eliminate unqualified experts. It's fair to expect an expert to know about at least three or four of these articles:

➤ Barber and Lucas (1983) *System Response Time, Operator Productivity, and Job Satisfaction* (Delays damage productivity. They also hurt workers' morale.)

➤ Beatty (1979) *Performance Effects of System Response Time in Human/Computer Tasks*

➤ Bergman (1981) *System Response Time and Problem Solving Behavior* (Delays hamper attempts to solve problems.)

➤ Gibson (1990) *Application Response Time Is Critical to Productivity*

➤ Rivera (1992) *An Empirical Study of the Effect of System Response Time and task Complexity on User Decision Quality* (Delays cause the most harm to the most complex tasks.)

➤ Stein (1983) *Relation Between User Think Time and Response Time in an Interactive System* (Users forget parts of tasks and must rethink them when system response time increases. This causes total thinking time to increase.)

➤ University of Utrecht (1982) *The Influence of System Response Time and Memory Load on Problem-Solving Behavior* (The more facts that users have to remember to solve a problem, the worse is the effect of computer system delays.)

⇨ Computer tasks that still take too long

Nowadays almost everything you do with a computer takes long enough to keep you from reaching your potential. Here are a few of the things that slow you down:

➤ Starting your computer

➤ Waiting for an application to launch

➤ Being unable to stop an application from launching after it starts

➤ Uploading or downloading files

➤ Screen scrolls

➤ Output

➤ Waiting for menus and dialog boxes to appear

- Searching for menu items and selecting them

- Waiting for find-and-replace operations to finish

- Waiting for mail-merges to finish

- Using a mouse or trackball to move a cursor

- And much, much more

It takes far longer than 0.3 seconds to reach for a mouse and use it to guide a cursor to a new position. Using a mouse is a complicated process. First, you must make a series of comparisons between the position of your hand and the position of the mouse, until your hand reaches the mouse. Then you must make fine adjustments to position the mouse in your hand properly. Having done this, you're still not done. You must now compare the position of the screen cursor with the position of a screen target, and move the cursor until it reaches the target. Chances are good that you will overshoot the screen target and have to back up and try again (real estate on today's computer displays is scarce, and targets are small). And if this is not bad enough, your mouse's trackball may have an eyelash or some lint wrapped around it, making it take an extra-long time for you to move the cursor to your target. So, using a mouse or trackball will take long enough to interrupt you almost every time you use it.

As you have already seen, delays that are longer that 0.3 seconds will hurt your productivity. So faster input devices will someday replace mice and trackballs, just as mice and trackballs replaced (some) keyboard entry.

How computer system delays reduce your productivity

Do you have a hobby so interesting it makes you lose all track of time? Have you ever been so firmly focused on your work that you were surprised when someone said it was lunch time? Do you often feel a deep sense of satisfaction with what you are doing, coupled with a loss of any sense that time is passing?

None of this happens when you use a slow computer system that makes you wait, does it? This is because slow computers interrupt your thought processes, forcing you to rethink tasks that you should only have to think about once. This is frustrating and inefficient.

The reason why you have to rethink tasks, after you have been interrupted, is that interruptions make you forget what you were doing when you were interrupted. Your short-term memory can hold only about seven different items of information at one time, plus or minus two items (Miller 1956). If an interruption forces you to turn to a new line of thought, this new line of thought will have to use your short-term memory. To do this you will have to flush some old items of information from your short-term memory. Your memory will replace some (or all) of these old items with new items that are related to your new line of thought. All of this will happen no matter what the interruption may be: getting a telephone call, overhearing a conversation, or using a computer that interrupts you because it cannot keep up with the speed of your thoughts.

Why should a computer delay of only 0.3 seconds matter so much? The reason is that a delay of 0.3 seconds can interrupt a great deal of mental activity and force you to rethink all of it. For example, your short-term memory can change its state every 0.001 to 0.005 seconds (Brady 1986). Thus, your short-term memory can change its state as many as 300 times during a 0.3-second computer delay. Making a simple decision may take you 0.01 seconds. More complex decisions may take you 0.075 seconds. So a 0.3-second computer delay wastes time that you might otherwise use to make four complex decisions. Worse than this, delays force you to spend additional thinking time re-establishing interrupted trains of thought, like having to find your place in a book that you accidentally dropped on the floor.

How much additional thinking time does it take for you to re-establish an interrupted train of thought? Doherty and Keliskey (1979) found that, after 15 seconds of computer system delay, each additional second of delay adds an additional second of thinking time. Shorter delays will add proportionally more thinking time.

⇨ Tasks that are damaged by computer delays

As you've already seen in Chapter 11, large capital expenditures for office equipment during the 1970s and 1980s brought little increase in the productivity of white-collar workers. At the same time, each new increase in computer speed has brought big increases in the productivity of computer programmers. How can both of these statements be true?

During the 1970s and 1980s, computer programmers spent a much larger proportion of their time using computers than other white-collar workers did. In marked contrast with other white-collar work, almost all of programmer's work was computerized. Compared with programmers, other white-collar workers had few computerized tools to use, so a smaller proportion of their work benefited from using computers.

The sudden increase in the productivity of white-collar workers that has been visible during the 1990s (seen partly as mass layoffs of middle managers) has happened because white-collar workers use computers for a bigger proportion of their work than they did before 1990. Now computer speed, as well as computer delays, affect everyone.

Computer delays (i.e., long computer system response times) reduce the productivity of workers who are doing tasks as simple as data entry. These delays decrease productivity of data entry workers even when they are highly experienced (Butler 1982).

Computer delays will reduce the productivity of workers whose jobs range in complexity from data entry to computer programming.

⇨ How you can boost the speed of your computer system

Luckily for you, there are many ways for you to increase the speed of your computer system. You can more than double your productivity,

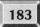

compared with using an average computer system, if you choose the right combination of hardware and software.

⇨ Hardware tips for increasing speed

Here are some hardware features that will give you some of the speed that you need:

➢ Faster printer, with more than eight megabytes of printer RAM

➢ Faster microprocessor (the fastest one available)

➢ Microprocessor cache, with at least 256 kilobytes of fast RAM

➢ Larger, faster computer RAM

➢ Multiprocessor computer, coupled with a symmetric multiprocessing operating system

➢ Numeric co-processor

➢ Faster computer expansion bus (PCI for graphics adapters and ISA for add-ons)

➢ Video accelerator board

➢ Larger, faster video cache

➢ 17-inch (or larger) video monitor for displaying several applications simultaneously

➢ Large, fast hard disk (size: 1GB or more, with access time less than 12 milliseconds)

➢ Larger, faster RAM disk

➢ Faster CD-ROM drive coupled with a 16-bit sound card that has wavetable sound synthesis

➢ Faster modem

⇨ Software tips for increasing speed

Avoid using data-compression software. Using it is a false economy because it cuts your hard disk speed. Buy a bigger hard disk instead,

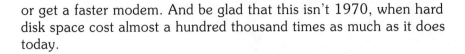

or get a faster modem. And be glad that this isn't 1970, when hard disk space cost almost a hundred thousand times as much as it does today.

Use a hard-disk-defragmentation utility. You'll be glad that you do, because it will seem as if you have next month's hard disk today.

Even if you work alone, a true multitasking system will boost your productivity. For one thing, you can more easily launch a different application if you change your mind about what you want to do. You won't have to wait for an unwanted application to finish launching before you can start a new one. And, of course, you'll be able to switch to a new application quickly instead of waiting for a lengthy task to complete. This way, you will be able to work more quickly, in a less linear style, and respond more quickly to changing circumstances. Be sure to use a large video monitor with your multitasking operating system.

If your computer is connected with a local-area network (LAN), the LAN should, of course, have a performance measuring system. The performance measuring system should look for network response times that exceed either of two predetermined thresholds. One threshold, the lowest one, should warn a network manager to begin taking corrective action. The other, higher, threshold should warn a network manager when network response time is slow enough to damage users' productivity.

If you're thinking about getting a local area network for the first time, you should, of course, get an LAN tuning system that lets you tune your LAN for speed, and adjust LAN parameters in response to warnings about LAN performance.

You can also boost your productivity by choosing software that offers you the most rapid response time. The following chapters tell you how to choose fast software. They tell you what software features you can and *should* have, while still having a fast computer system. They also tell you how to optimize your computer system to get the most from this software.

Choosing software for writing & desktop publishing

CHOOSING the fastest possible word processor is probably the best way for you to boost your productivity, and the productivity of anyone who works for you. That's because word processing accounts for 85 percent of all personal computer use, a proportion that has not changed in 15 years (Schwabach 1993).

If you, or anyone who works for you, do a lot of writing, and you want to control how things look in print, you need to get desktop publishing software. Whatever else you do, make sure it is fast.

Word processing

You'll need to consider both hardware and software when you choose the fastest possible computer system for word processing.

Hardware tips

Make sure your computer system has these hardware features:

> ➤ Fast printer, with lots of high-speed printer RAM
> ➤ Fast microprocessor
> ➤ Eight megabytes of computer RAM
> ➤ Fast computer bus
> ➤ Video accelerator board
> ➤ High-speed hard disk

Software tips

When you choose a word processor you should pay special attention to the speed with which you can:

> ➤ Launch the word processor
> ➤ Scroll screens
> ➤ Fetch and store files

➢ Select text

➢ Find and replace text

➢ Move text

➢ Copy text

➢ Delete text

➢ Print files

➢ Change type fonts and type sizes

➢ Move the cursor

⇨ Ease of use

You need to consider ease of use, in addition to speed. Look for easy-to-use:

➢ Text & page-layout features

➢ User interface

➢ Command strategies

➢ Disk and memory-usage efficiency

➢ Text entry and editing facilities

➢ Grammar and hyphenation capability

➢ Interactive table editing capability

➢ Math facilities

➢ Graphics facilities

➢ Data export/import facilities

➢ Document creation capabilities

➢ Dynamic data linking capability

➢ Printing ease

❋ **Text & page layout**

The text and page-layout features of your word processor should include style sheets that change text formats automatically, kerning (adjustable letter spacing), automatic adjustment of line spacing in relation to font size, and widows and orphans control. Your word processor should be able to keep designated paragraphs together. It should be possible for you to set conditional page breaks. Vertical centering should be automatic.

The word processor should also be able to convert nonprinting comments to text.

❋ **User interface**

The screen display should have rulers that can be displayed or suppressed. Screens should display margins and tabs, too. Screens should have a format ribbon for choosing text and font attributes. The word processor should also support what-you-see-is-what-you-get (WYSIWYG) editing.

The word processor should support text wrapping and print and graphics preview, and it should show page breaks and paragraph markers.

❋ **Command strategy**

The word processor's command strategy should include both command line control and a mouse-controlled, menu-driven interface. It should format text by inserting codes in files.

❋ **Text entry & editing**

Your word processor should have text entry and editing features that are powerful and easy to use. These features should include numerous undo levels. Choose a word processor that lets you search-and-replace text by using wild cards. Your word processor should also allow case-sensitive searches and it should recognize whole words. It should be able to search for (and replace) fonts, text attributes, formats, and nonstandard characters.

✳ Grammar & hyphenation

Your word processor's hyphenation and grammar utilities should be able to spellcheck single words or defined blocks as you type. It should be able to hyphenate words on-the-fly, using either algorithms or a dictionary. It should also have an integrated grammar checker and a thesaurus.

✳ Interactive table editor

Choose a word processor that has an interactive table editor. Make sure it lets you continue tables past page breaks and put graphics in table cells. Also make sure it lets you put dynamic functions in tables.

✳ Math facilities

It is often convenient to be able to put mathematical functions in documents, so choose a word processor that can do this. Its math facilities should also include a keyboard calculator.

✳ Graphics

Your word processor should be able to flow text around documents, draw lines by using a mouse or other input device, insert drawings in the flow of text, import drawings and resize them by using a mouse, use menus to insert lines, and display graphics by using an equation editor.

✳ Data export/import

Your word processor's file manager should be able to import/export many data formats, including .BMP, .CDL, .CGM, .DRW, EPS, HPGL, .MSP, .PCX, .PIC, TIFF, WMF, and .WPG.

✳ Document creation

Your word processor's document-creation capabilities should include automatic creation of tables of contents and automatic creation of indexes that have multiple levels. It should make it easy for you to create cross-references and it should automatically number endnotes and footnotes. You should be able to make collapsible outlines that have customizable numbering.

✳ **Dynamic data links**

Your word processor should let you create documents that have dynamic links to spreadsheets and other software. They should also be able to use client/server OLE support, and it should also be possible for your documents to have text-file links.

✳ **Printing**

Support for printing is a key feature. It should include background printing, using a print queue that can be modified. Your word processor should be able to print the current page, defined blocks of pages, and discontinuous ranges of pages. It should also be able to collate a print job, format envelopes and labels, and print both landscape and portrait pages in the same run. Finally, your word processor's print facility should be able to print files from a file-manager list.

⇨ Desktop publishing software

When you choose a system for desktop publishing you need to consider both hardware and software, just as you did when you chose a system for word processing.

⇨ Hardware tips

Your computer system needs the same hardware optimization for desktop publishing that it needs for word processing. In addition, you'll need a larger hard disk than you need for word processing, especially if you must handle many images.

You should also have a removable hard disk if you take material to a service bureau or send it back and forth to a publisher. Remember that removable hard disks are more fragile than fixed ones, so don't try to use one as your primary hard disk.

⇨ Software tips

Your desktop publishing software needs to be strong in six key areas: fonts and typography; text handling; document layout; graphics handling; output; and platform and network support.

✳ Fonts and typography

Your desktop publishing program should support HP cartridge fonts, TrueType, Agfa Intellifonts, and Bitstream Speedo. Ligatures and kerning should be automatic, but it should be possible for you to define tracking, edit kerning and tracking tables, and adjust baselines. You should be able to select type from a large range of type fonts and point sizes. You should also be able to rotate type.

✳ Text handling

Text handling should include automatic creation of bulleted lists and search-and-replacement of special characters, nonprinting characters, regular characters, and named styles, including character styles and section styles. It should be easy to remove bullets from bulleted lists.

The text handling facility should support vertical alignment and justification. It should also support conditional text. The text handler should be able to import style sheets as well as text formats such as DCA/RTF, WordPerfect, Microsoft Word, and WordStar. It should also be possible to import such data formats as .DBF and .WK?/.XLS.

Finally, the text-handling facility should include a spellchecker, a table editor, and an equation editor.

✳ Document layout

Your desktop publishing program's document-layout features should include thumbnail displays that you can use to rearrange pages. Its document-layout features should include support for section numbering and page numbering. Text-alignment options should include freeform guides and independent x and y rulers. Maximum page size should be at least 48×48 inches. It should be possible to have several dozen master pages for each document. There should be no limit to the number of pages per document, and there should be no limit to the number of columns. There should be lock frames, too.

✳ Graphics handling

Graphics handling should include tools for drawing Bezier and freehand curves, as well as polygons and polylines. You should be able to wrap text around irregularly shaped graphics and within a nonrectangular graphic frame. Graphic frame shapes should include rectangles, circles, and ellipses, as well as regular and irregular polygons.

You should be able to flip, mirror, or rotate objects. You should also be able to assemble and disassemble groups of objects.

Color handling should include use of fill patterns, user specification of tints, and support for a wide variety of color models. These color models should include RGB, CMYK, Pantone, TrueMatch, Focoltone, HSB, and HLS.

Graphics handling should include the ability to import .BMP (DIB), .DRW (Micrografx), .DXF, HPGL, EPS, DCS, .PCX, Intel TIFF, Motorola TIFF, and .WPG (WordPerfect Graphic). You should, of course, be able to edit bitmap graphics.

✳ Output

Output support should include the ability to create process-color separations, with black generation and specification of color channel frequencies and angles. It should be possible to use an unlimited number of spot colors and convert spot colors to CMYK.

Users should be able to trap to or from any color, specify halftone dot shape, angle, and frequency, and do overprints and knockouts. Users should also be able to print negatives that have registration marks and steps scales.

✳ Platform & network support

Desktop publishing software should support DDE and OLE clients. It should support file locking and should allow users to share documents and templates.

14

Choosing database, document, & contact management software

NOT everyone uses database software, but if you do you should choose the fastest database software you can get. And you should optimize your computer system so it gives you the best possible speed.

Optimization for general database software, including relational database software, is also applicable to more specialized database software, including software for managing documents and personal contacts.

⇨ Relational database software

You'll need to optimize both your hardware and your software when you choose a new database package. Here is how to do it.

⇨ Hardware tips

If you plan to do a lot of database work, make sure your computer system has these features:

> ➢ Fast microprocessor

> ➢ More than eight megabytes of RAM

> ➢ Numeric co-processor

> ➢ Fast computer bus

> ➢ Large, very-high-speed hard disk

> ➢ RAM disk

See Chapter 12 for more details about hardware optimization.

If your database is large and heavily used by many users, you should have a multiprocessor computer, coupled with an appropriate operating system.

Software tips

When you choose a database package, pay special attention to these aspects of the package:

➢ Application development language

➢ Application development facilities

➢ Data type

➢ Data limits

➢ Data definition and integrity procedures

➢ Data importing and exporting facilities

➢ Data querying capability

➢ Indexing

➢ Multi-user capability

➢ Security facilities

The database features that will have the biggest impact on your speed and productivity are its application development language, application development facilities, data querying facilities, and indexing methods.

✳ Application development language

Choose a relational database that offers a compiled language, not an interpreted one. Your applications will run faster if you do. It's also a good idea to choose a package that supports SQL. Finally, choose a database package that can create macros automatically, by monitoring your keystrokes. This will save you endless time spent in debugging macros.

✳ Application development facilities

Your relational database should be able to generate applications, menus, and reports. You shouldn't have to program these from scratch, unless you have unusual requirements. You'll be more productive if your new database package also includes built-in facilities for debugging applications.

✳ Data types

Choose a database that should support arrays of many data types, including:

- ➤ Dimensional
- ➤ Variable-Length
- ➤ Fixed-Character
- ➤ Variable-Character
- ➤ Integer
- ➤ Fixed-Decimal
- ➤ Floating-Point decimal
- ➤ Date
- ➤ Time
- ➤ Boolean

✳ Data limits

The maximum size of columns or fields should be at least 256 characters. The maximum size of rows or records should be at least 4K, but 64K is better. Nowadays, some database packages offer unlimited fields per record, but a limit of 255 fields is typical. Some databases offer an unlimited number of indexed fields per record but, again, a limit of 255 is typical.

Several database packages for personal computers support an unlimited number of records per table or file, but a million records is more common. Most database packages support an unlimited number of files or tables per database. They also support an unlimited number of indexes per database.

✳ Data definition and integrity procedures

Some database packages support data dictionaries, but you can get along without them. Some database packages support file catalogs, too, but you don't really need one of these, either. You do need a robust facility for data validation, including data-type enforcement, pattern matching, specification of data ranges, table lookups, soundex matching, rule-based matching, and user-definable rules for matching. Your database package should also support composite keys and should require primary keys.

✳ Data importing and exporting facilities

Your database package should let you import or export numerous standard file formats, including ASCII (fixed-length, tab-delimited, and comma-delimited), .DBF/.DIF, .PFS/.SDF, .WK1/.WKQ, and .XLS/SYLK.

You should be able to define file formats of your own.

✳ Data querying capability

Your database package should include a query language that is compatible with SQL. It should have a query interface that supports queries by example and queries by form. You'll get more productivity in the beginning if the query interface is controlled by menus or dialog boxes, not command lines. But you will have to pay for this convenience and the easy learning curve later, unless the query interface lets you do things both ways.

If your database package can precompile and optimize queries, it will execute them faster. Querying should support nested (recursive) queries. It should be possible for you to sort on any field or on any combination of fields. Ideally, the number of search fields should be unlimited.

These are the relational operators that a query facility should support:

➢ Difference (MINUS)

➢ Divide (DIVIDEBY)

➢ Intersect

➢ Join (natural and outer)

➤ Project

➤ Product (TIMES)

➤ Select (WHERE)

➤ Union

✳ Indexing

Your database package should support such indexing and access methods as b-trees, clustered b-trees, and hashing. Insist on a database package that has automatic indexing that you can turn on or off. It should support composite indexes, too.

You should be able to define an exclusion list. Your database package should also support uniques, and should let you index keys.

✳ Multi-User capability

If you are choosing a database package for a multi-user environment, make sure it supports three kinds of locks: coordinated, exclusive and shared. Your database package should be able to lock indexes, fields, records, files, and databases. It should also be able to identify stations that have locks activated.

Multi-user transaction processing should include transaction definition, implicit locking, and commit/rollback, including a two-phase commit.

The database package should support time-out and retry control procedures. It should support NetWare networks, Vines, Unix, and, maybe, Microsoft LAN manager.

✳ Security facilities

Your database package should support application encryption and data encryption. You should be able to extend password protection to databases, data dictionaries, fields, records, tables, users, and groups of users.

Ideally, your database package should be able to provide user-specific interfaces and should restrict the use of commands.

⇨ Document management software

These are the key features that you should look at when you choose document management software:

- ➤ Document management features
- ➤ Data import/export facilities
- ➤ Indexing & sorting facilities
- ➤ Search facilities
- ➤ Document retrieval facilities
- ➤ Reporting facilities
- ➤ Administration and security
- ➤ Vendor support

Document management software should also have a high-quality database engine and convenient archiving and de-archiving facilities.

⇨ Document management features

The document management software package that you choose should, of course, have a wide range of functions that are purely for document management. These should include document logging, version tracking, document relocation ability, automatic file naming, the ability to make documents private or public, and a facility for assigning filenames.

⇨ Data import/export facilities

Your document management package should allow bulk importing and importing into specified fields. It should support these data formats: ASCII (fixed-length, tab-delimited, and comma-delimited), .DBF, Microsoft Word for Windows files, WordPerfect files, .WK?, and .XLS.

Indexing and sorting facilities

Choose a document management package that has fast, strong indexing and sorting capabilities. It should be able to index by such fields as:

> Author

> Creation date

> Current date

> Document category

> Document number

> Full text, keywords

> Schedule, subject

> Any user-defined category

It should be possible for you to sort on primary fields, any other fields, or by multiple fields.

Search facilities

Your document manager needs to have a database engine for searching data for profiles. The engine should be able to search full text. It should be possible for you to do transparent searches, locally and across networks. It should also be possible for you to use search operators such as AND, OR, exclusive OR, NOT, > (greater than), < (less than), and not equal.

It is best if you can do searches by combining a large number of these operators. Your document manager should let you search by author, client, date of document creation, date range, document number, or user-defined categories.

It should be possible for you to search full text, search for profiles, or combine searches of full text with searches for profiles. Also, you should be able to use fuzzy logic, nested searches, pattern matching, phonetic searching (Soundex), querying by example, and wild-card searches.

⇨ Document retrieval facilities

Your document management software should let you view ASCII files, files from AmiPro, Lotus 1-2-3, Lotus 1-2-3 for Windows, Microsoft Excel, Microsoft Word for Windows, Quattro Pro, and WordPerfect. It should be possible for you to view bitmapped graphics files as well as vector graphics files of all kinds. In addition, your document management software should let you use document viewers produced by third parties.

⇨ Reporting facilities

Your document management software should let you create customized reports. Its reporting facility should also include pre-defined reports, for example, document storage maps, and reports that list files that have been archived, deleted, or accessed.

Your document management software should be able to purge documents automatically by author, client, date, subject, and other fields. It should be possible for you to have reports exported to other software. Finally, reporting facilities should be able to describe user and system configurations and report any configuration changes.

⇨ Administration & security

The document manager should use Novell NetWare security. It should also provide its own security. It should be able to encrypt documents. Access permission should be assignable to individual users, to groups, to specific directories, or to specific documents or categories of documents. Users should be able to prevent others from viewing profiles.

Administration and security facilities should keep a log of all accesses and attempted accesses to the document management system. The document manager should also be able to establish access levels, including no access, read filenames only, read files only, and write access. These access levels should be assignable to individuals or to groups.

⇨ Vendor support

Vendor support should include context-sensitive help, on-line help, toll-free technical support, a vendor-supported BBS, and printed documentation.

⇨ Contact management software

Contact management software packages handle associations between people. They are distinguished from personal information management software (PIMs) in that PIMs are concerned with a sequence of activities that usually are connected to a database of addresses and schedules.

⇨ Hardware tips

Optimize your contact management software the same way you would optimize a general-purpose database package. In addition, make sure that the modems you use are fast. See Chapter 12 and the beginning of this chapter for more details about hardware optimization.

⇨ Software tips

The most important criteria for choosing contact management software are its:

➤ Databa.e features

➤ Querying facilities

➤ Data import/export facilities

➤ Telephone call automation

➤ Telephone call history recording

➤ Scheduling facilities

➤ Word processing capabilities

➤ Faxing facilities

➤ Reports & utilities

➤ Vendor support

✳ **Database features**

It should be easy for you to insert information in fields, using dialog boxes or customizable data lists. You should also be able to enter, duplicate, or remove records easily.

You should be able to define a large number of fields, at least 100. Pre-defined fields should include fields for e-mail carrier, fax number, contact name, and customer ID.

Ideally, there should be a large, possibly unlimited, number of telephone numbers for each contact. The number of alternative contacts should be unlimited, too. The maximum number of fields per record, records per database, and databases should be unlimited.

✳ **Querying facilities**

Contact management software should be able to index user-defined fields or pre-defined fields such as company name, first name, last name, city, state, zip code, phone number, and contact type.

You should be able to define subsets of contacts and conduct Boolean searches of these and other subsets. You should be able to search freeform text fields, search multiple fields, and save the results of your queries.

✳ **Data import/export**

Contact management software should be able to import/export ASCII files (fixed-length, comma-delimited, or tab-delimited), and import from or export to other contact management software. You should be able to detect and remove duplicate entries.

✳ **Telephone call automation**

Telephone call automation should include automatic re-dialing, local area-code dialing prefix adjustment, and global dialing prefix adjustment.

✳ **Telephone call history recording**

Contact management software should time- and date-stamp telephone calls, and should record the last action taken (for all fields). Contact management software should also issue periodic follow-up reminders.

Users should be able to purge history files selectively, for example, by date of call.

✳ **Scheduling facilities**

Scheduling is, of course, a key feature of contact management software. The scheduling facility should include a calendar with an adjustable time scale. It should offer users a weekly view, a monthly view, and a yearly view of scheduled activities.

Users should be able to assign priority levels to tasks. A tickler file function should be able to buzz an event alarm within other software applications.

Users should be able to attach notes to tasks. Unfinished tasks should be carried forward from current lists.

✳ **Word processing**

Contact management software needs to have an integrated word processor. It should have links to external word processors and should include a spellchecker.

The word processing facility should have an integrated mail merge facility, a letter generator, and the ability to import boilerplate text. Users should be able to print envelopes and labels.

✳ **Faxes**

Contact management software should be able to send or receive faxes, using delayed transmission if necessary. It should be able to fax boilerplate text and queue faxes for multiple faxing.

15

Choosing software for accounting & analyzing numbers

HIGH-SPEED accounting and spreadsheet software can yield a big payoff, especially if it is on a network. Slow software on the network gives the same productivity problems that you've already read about in Chapter 12, in connection with timesharing systems.

⇨ Spreadsheets

As in other situations you need to optimize both hardware and software to get the fastest spreadsheet action. Here is how to do it.

⇨ Hardware tips

It's useful to think of a spreadsheet as database software that has extra requirements for calculating results and creating graphics. So, you should optimize your system the same as you would optimize it for a general-purpose database. Additionally, you should have a high-speed math co-processor and a video accelerator card installed in your computer (see Chapters 12 and 14 for more details about hardware optimization).

⇨ Software tips

The most important features to consider when you choose a spreadsheet are:

➤ Auditing facilities

➤ Data import/export

➤ Data capacity

➤ Database facilities

➤ Data analysis

➤ Recalculation

➤ Formatting

➤ Publishing

➢ Charts and graphs

➢ Text-file support

➢ Macros

➢ Model building

➢ Printing

➢ Security

➢ Hardware support

Your productivity will be greater if you choose a spreadsheet that does data analysis, recalculation, and data import and export at high speed, because these are key spreadsheet features that you will use almost all the time. You should also make sure your spreadsheet can make charts and graphs and print results at high speed.

✳ Auditing facilities

Your spreadsheet's auditing features should include a map mode, text annotation of formulas (as attached notes), and annotation by means of text boxes that are attached to drawing layers. Spreadsheets should also be able to use sound to annotate formulas.

You should be able to display the antecedents and consequents of formulas. You should also be able to trace through all of the elements of a circular reference chain.

✳ Data import/export

Your spreadsheet should have Lotus 1-2-3 file compatibility. It should also be able to import or export files with these formats:

.DB	.WK1
.DBF	.WK3
.DIF	.WQ1
.SLK	.WR1
.WB1	.XLS 3.x
.WKS	.XLS 4.0

✳ Data capacity

Nowadays you can get spreadsheets that have enormous data capacity. Some spreadsheets will let you open an unlimited number of files. Others will support thousands of rows and hundreds of columns and pages.

✳ Database facilities

Choose a spreadsheet that lets you develop customized data entry screens in addition to the ready-made data entry screens that it supplies. Make sure that your spreadsheet can search-and-replace data, too.

Other database features that you can reasonably expect to have are the ability to sort by row or column, using many sort keys, and the ability to query external database files, join two database tables, or do frequency analyses, using commands and functions.

✳ Data analysis

At a minimum you can expect to have functions for math, date and time, statistics, finance, string manipulation, logic, and database statistics. And you should be able to create your own custom functions, too, though some spreadsheets offer libraries functions. These can save you lots of development time.

Sooner or later you may want to do matrix manipulations and linear regression, too. Nowadays most popular spreadsheets let you do these operations.

✳ Recalculation

Make sure that your spreadsheet has natural recalculation abilities, intelligent recalculation abilities, and manual recalculation abilities. You should also make sure that it can do automatic recalculation in the background. If it can do recalculation as a background activity, it will save you lots of time and will interrupt your work less often.

✳ Formatting

Choose a spreadsheet that lets you create named styles, define numeric formats, create custom currency symbols, and name and reuse font sets. The ability to create named styles will save you time.

Your spreadsheet should display negative amounts in parentheses, and should align currency symbols and parentheses. It should be able to display numbers as left-justified or as centered. Make sure that it can display the text of formulas cell by cell or throughout an entire spreadsheet, with the text of these formulas properly centered, too.

Your spreadsheet's displays should be able to use shading and color. For example, it should be possible for its color choices to depend on the values of the numbers that are being displayed. It should be able to use scalable fonts and bitmapped fonts. These fonts should include italic and bold face as well as normal type faces. It should be possible for you to use several type fonts per worksheet.

In addition to text and numbers, your spreadsheet should be able to display geometric shapes via a separate drawing layer. It should be possible for you to embed graphics on the worksheet, too.

✳ Publishing

It should be easy to create reports that have line drawings and borders, multiline labels, and label text that is oriented vertically or horizontally.

✳ Charts and graphs

Almost any spreadsheet that you choose will support an unlimited number of points per series, series per chart, and points per chart. Make sure that the one that you choose lets you specify a multiple series as a single range. Your spreadsheet should also be able to parse series of points, based on the shape of the range.

Choose a spreadsheet that supports both two-dimensional charts and three-dimensional charts. Two-dimensional charts should include:

> ➤ Vertical bar

> ➤ Stacked vertical bar

> ➤ Horizontal bar

> ➤ Line

> ➤ X/Y

> Area

> Pie charts

> Multi-series pie charts

> Pie-bar

> Radar

> High-low-close

> High-low-close-open

> Text charts

> Combinations of all these

Three-dimensional charts should include 3-D vertical bar, vertical bar with each series in its own plane, line (ribbon), area, pie, and surface or wireframe charts.

You should be able to specify the intersections of chart axes, suppress any axis or grid lines, scale axes logarithmically, scale axes manually, and adjust the space between bar markers. You should also be able to annotate individual chart points with arrows or freehand drawings, or floating text.

Choose a spreadsheet that lets you customize data-point markers with borders and gradient fills. You will also find it very useful to be able to replace standard markers with bitmaps, and to assign scaling factors to data point labels. Nowadays you can count on being able to get a spreadsheet that can stagger these labels automatically. You can also count on getting one that lets you customize chart backgrounds, replacing them with bitmaps, or adding 3-D chart rotation, elevation, or perspective.

❊ **Text file support**

You'll find it very useful to be able to import and export tab-delimited files, comma-delimited files, and files with user-defined delimiters. Nowadays most spreadsheets let you do this.

✳ Macros

Insist on a spreadsheet that has a macro recorder that can watch your actions and automatically create corresponding macros. This will save you no end of trouble debugging macros—you'll hardly have to debug such macros at all.

Your spreadsheet should also support event-triggered macros such as auto-load and auto-close. Also, make sure that your spreadsheet lets you use macros to create custom menus and custom dialog boxes.

Look for such macro debugging facilities as single-step tracing, conditional breakpoints, and watch variables.

Your spreadsheet's macros should be able to operate on external files or execute DOS commands. Its macro facility should have an interface to low-level languages such as C or C++. Finally, it should let you use macro libraries that are independent of worksheets.

✳ Model building

Your spreadsheet's model-building tools should let you build true 3-D worksheets. You should be able to hide rows, columns, worksheets or windows. You should also be able to open two or more windows that can be moved independently, split the screen horizontally or vertically, and drag and drop objects from place to place.

Choose a spreadsheet that lets you freeze rows and columns as titles, set column width for widest entry or set column height for tallest entry, and do partial-column or partial-row insertions or deletions. It should also let you create named associations of 2-D spreadsheets, and create named scenarios.

Your spreadsheet's model-building and editing facility should include an outliner, a spellchecker, and an Undo command, as well as a command to repeat the last action. It should be able to group-edit. It should be able to copy and erase formats.

✳ Printing

The spreadsheet program's print previewer should let users adjust margins and column widths. It should also let them specify scaling factors and starting page numbers.

Spreadsheet printing should be done in the background. Printing should be possible in either portrait or landscape mode, with or without cell grid lines, and with or without worksheet frames. The spreadsheet printing facility should be able to print multiline headers and footers, and use worksheet ranges as headings.

Users should be able to create named libraries of print settings. And finally, users should be able to print the text of formulas, each on a separate line.

✳ Security

Your spreadsheet program should support timed backup, done in the background. It should warn you against overwrite by a save operation, and create a backup file during each save operation, in case anything goes wrong. Your spreadsheet program also should be able to protect files with a password system, and should be able to lock or hide the contents of worksheet cells.

✳ Hardware support

Make sure that your spreadsheet program supports a math co-processor. It should also be available on multiple platforms.

⇨ LAN-Based accounting software

Optimize your combination of hardware and LAN-based accounting software in much the same way that you would optimize a system for single-user accounting software (see Chapters 12 and 14 for more details).

⇨ Hardware tips

If your business is large, consider using a multiprocessor computer, plus a multitasking operating system.

⇨ Software tips

These are the key areas for you to consider when you choose a LAN-based accounting package:

➤ Enterprise scale

➤ Customization

➤ General ledger

➤ Accounts payable

➤ Accounts receivable

➤ Inventory

➤ Order entry

➤ Purchase order

✳ Enterprise scale

The size of your firm matters when you are choosing LAN-based accounting software. The criteria listed here are for firms that have annual revenues between $500,000 and $50 million dollars. If your company's sales are less than $500,000 a year you probably don't need LAN-based accounting software. On the other hand, if your sales are more than $50 million, you may want to have an accounting system customized by an accounting firm.

✳ Customization

Customization capabilities should include a macro facility, preferably one that can make macros automatically by noting what you do and recording your keystrokes. It should be possible for each user of your accounting system to have a customized menu, different data-entry field names, and different lookup windows. Vendors should also make source code available to you.

✳ General ledger

The general ledger module of your accounting package should support intercompany postings, perform allocations and multicurrency conversions, and be capable of multicurrency transactions that comply with FASB-52. It should be possible for you to produce statistical accounts and multiple retained earnings accounts. You should be able to handle more than 100 budgets per accounting period.

✳ **Accounts payable**

LAN-based accounts payable modules should be able to flag 1099 items by line item. You should be able to post intercompany vouchers and customize checks. Your accounting package should be able to allocate at least eight alphanumeric characters to a vendor number.

Accounts payable modules should be able to do multicurrency transactions. You should be able to calculate commissions based on payments received, or on gross profits.

✳ **Order entry**

Your accounting system's order entry module should let you order items by using your customer's part numbers. It should also be able to handle drop shipments, and should be able to track customer request dates as line items.

✳ **Inventory**

Inventory modules should report slow-moving or obsolete items, price items by customer class or by product class, and should track items by serial number or by lot number. The maximum number of levels in a bill of materials should be at least ten.

Inventory modules should support an unlimited number of FIFO levels. They should support average, standard, and last inventory costing methods. Users should be able to produce reorder reports for each warehouse. They should be able to track unit costs by stocking locations and define costing methods at the item level. Inventory modules should allocate 20 alphanumeric characters to each item code.

✳ **Purchase order**

Purchase order modules should be able to perform multicurrency transactions. They should be able to create purchase orders automatically, using reorder information. They should also be able to process requisitions for materials.

⇨ Statistics software

Statistics software presents all of the optimization problems that you would encounter if you optimized a system for doing high-speed accounting, graphics, math, and database operations. So be sure to look again at Chapters 14 and 16.

✳ Hardware tips

Make sure you have a very high-speed math co-processor and a very high-speed microprocessor installed in your computer. Nowadays statistical packages do a lot of graphics work, so be sure you have a high-quality video accelerator board installed as well. See Chapter 12 for more details.

⇨ Software tips

Statistics software must be strong in the following areas:

> Data entry and editing

> Data management

> Table handling

> T-tests (univariate)

> Regression and designed experiments

> Analysis of variance

> Multi-variate analysis of variance

> Graphics

> Output

Choose a statistical package that has a procedural language and a report writer.

✳ **Data entry and editing**

Your statistical software should include a data editor. It should be able to import or export dBase, SQL, and .WK* files. It should be able to handle array data, grouped data sets, and hierarchical data sets.

The maximum number of data points and observations should be limited only by available hard disk space. Statistical software should also be able to handle thousands of different variables.

✳ **Data management**

Users should be able to select subsets of variables for analysis; for example, splitting files into two parts. They should also be able to select data conditionally, including on the basis of the range of variables. Of course, it's very important for users to be able to sort data in ascending or descending order, using numerous sort keys; for example, 10 or more at a time. They should be able to select data-transformation functions, using menus or dialog boxes. A spreadsheet interface should be available. Data management also should include facilities for using probability functions and inverse probability functions, and leading and lagging data.

✳ **Table handling**

Statistical software should be able to create stub-and-banner tables, as well as single, multiway tables. It should be able to compute chi-square tests of independence on tables, and as well as compute other tests of independence. It should also compute descriptive statistics for breakdown tables.

✳ **T-tests**

Choose statistical software that can compute t-tests, including t-tests for paired data.

✳ **Regression**

Your statistical software should be able to compute linear regression, nonlinear regression, censored regression, robust regression, and ridge regression. It should support generalized linear models (GLMs) and generalized co-variance structure analysis.

Linear regression should allow automatic selection of all possible data subsets. It should support standard multiple regression, weighted regression, and basic residuals analysis. Extended-regression diagnostics and co-linearity diagnostics should be available.

The facility for nonlinear regression should let users specify functions and derivatives. A derivative-free method should also be available. General, logistic, and probit nonlinear regression should be supported.

✳ Analysis of variance and experimental design

Statistical software packages should have complete facilities for performing ANOVAs (analyses of variance) and ANCOVAs (analyses of co-variance). They should also support factorial design specification, be able to perform post hoc tests, and do power analyses. Finally, they should support nested designs and be able to perform contrasts and planned comparisons.

✳ Multi-variate analysis of variance

The statistical package that you choose should be able to perform cluster analysis, discriminant analysis, and multidimensional scaling. It should also support principal components factor analysis. These analyses should yield factor scores. You should be able to rotate factor loadings and do confirmatory analyses.

Your package should include time-series procedures, functions for performing life-table analyses, and tests for quality control.

✳ Graphics

Your statistical package should support a wide range of graphics, including boxplots, histograms, line graphs, pie charts, scatterplots, 3-D graphs, and multidimensional graphics. Histograms should allow curve fitting. You should be able to make stem-and-leaf histograms, too. Your scatterplots should be able to show regression lines and least-square confidence bands. You should be able to make multiple plots on one page. Your statistical package should be able to make several different kinds of 3-D plots, including contour plots (ridge plots), general-function plots, point cloud rotation plots, projection-line plots, regression-plane plots, and spiked plots.

Make sure your statistical package lets you manipulate visual data interactively. Also, it should offer WYSIWYG chart editing.

✳ Output

You will want your output to look good, so make sure that the statistical package you choose supports a wide range of output devices, including laser printers, plotters, and color printers of all kinds.

16

Choosing software for handling images & sound

S OFTWARE for handling images and sound is becoming increasingly important. Chances are good that you—or someone who works for you—will be using multimedia authoring software, presentation software, desktop presentation software, and other graphics software, including software for screen capture and conversion, 24-bit paint programs, 2-D drafting programs, image editing software, and illustration programs.

⇨ Hardware tips

If you use graphics software your computer should have a high-quality video accelerator card, a math co-processor and a very high-speed microprocessor. Ideally, you should have a multiprocessor computer if you can afford it. And you need the best possible CD-ROM drive and sound card.

⇨ Multimedia authoring software

Here are the key areas for you to consider when you choose a multimedia authoring package:

- ➤ Developer interface
- ➤ Programming facilities
- ➤ Data formats
- ➤ Data importing and exporting
- ➤ Device synchronization
- ➤ Graphics facilities
- ➤ Sound
- ➤ Text
- ➤ Video
- ➤ User navigation

Pay special attention to user-navigation facilities, data importing and exporting methods, the developer interface, and programming facilities (unless you are an end user) when you choose a software for authoring multimedia. These features will have the largest impact on your productivity.

⇨ Developer interface

The developer interface of your multimedia authoring software should, of course be based on graphics, not text. It should incorporate a toolbox and ribbon bar. You should be able to hide menu bars and title bars to reduce screen clutter. It should also allow you to create icon flowcharts and nested flowcharts. You should be able to have multiple documents open and should be able to use zoom views to look at them.

It is useful for the developer interface to have password control that allows some users to have full authority to create and edit applications and lets others access and read only.

⇨ Programming facilities

Programming facilities should include a debugger. Multimedia authoring software should support arrays, integers, strings and user-defined variables.

You'll save development time if your multimedia authoring software is object-oriented. Its objects should include alphanumeric entry, checkboxes, dialog boxes, dragging and dropping, pull-down menus, push buttons and radio buttons. Finally, its programming facilities should offer you methods for timing and scoring.

⇨ Data formats

Multimedia authoring software should support these data file formats in ASCII (fixed-length, tab-delimited, or comma-delimited), dBase, and Q+E Database Library.

⇨ Data importing & exporting

Multimedia authoring software should be able to import a wide variety of data, including animations, graphics and sound. Animation formats that it should support are .FLC, .FLI and .MMM. The audio formats that it should support are CD audio, MIDI, .WAV and .SND. Graphics formats that it should support include .BMP, EPS, .GIF, .PCX, .PIC, PICT, .RLE, .TGA, TIFF, and .WMF.

⇨ Device synchronization

Multimedia authoring software should support event-driven timing. It should also support concurrent timing.

⇨ Graphics facilities

Graphics facilities should support 16.8 million colors, and you should be able to edit all these colors. There should be support for transition effects, animation, and video. Animation should include point-to-point, straight line or curved path, and simple cel animation. Video facilities should support QuickTime for Windows and Microsoft Video for Windows.

⇨ Sound

Sound should be able to loop repeatedly or until some triggering event occurs. It should be possible to kill sound when a new sound begins, when a triggering event occurs, or at any arbitrarily-chosen point.

⇨ Text

Text-handling facilities should support outline fonts. It should be possible for you to add drop shadows or frames, or perform rotation or sweeping. It should also be possible for you to extrude text, fit it to a curve, or bevel it.

Video

Multimedia authoring software should be able to drive a VCR or videodisk player. It should be able to run full-screen video as well as cropped video. It should support keyed overlays.

User navigation

Multimedia authoring software should support four kinds of navigation commands: jumps to beginning or end, GOTO commands, forward/backward, and dynamic hyperlinks.

Presentation software

Here are the areas to consider when you choose presentation software:

- Text charts
- Business charts
- Technical charts
- Data handling
- Chart editing and formatting
- Color handling
- Annotation
- Illustration
- Presentation management
- Electronic presentations
- Hard-copy presentations
- Vendor support

Data handling, chart creation, and editing and formatting are the three areas in which speed counts the most.

⇨ Text charts

Presentation graphics software should be able to justify text, adjust kerning and leading, adjust text on a baseline, set margins, and indent text or rotate it. It should be able to create multicolumn tables automatically. It should also be able to create text charts in stages.

The facility for creating text charts should support Adobe Type 1 and Type 2 typefaces, as well as Bitstream, Speedo, TrueType, Monotype, FaceLift, and Upgrade Systems. It should support the Adobe Type Manager, too. There should be no restrictions on the type formats supported.

The presentation software package should include a spellchecker for editing text charts.

⇨ Business charts

Business charts should include true 3-D bar and column charts, 2- and 3-D pie charts, cumulative-area charts, as well as bubble charts, Gantt charts, and organization charts. Other types of business charts should include line and scatter plots, high-low-open-close plots, and combination charts. Combination charts should include line over bar, line over area, and high-low over bar charts.

It should be possible for you to shadow and project 3-D column or bar charts, and have a choice between making them plain, stacked, overlapped or clustered.

The charting facility should be able to create proportional pie charts, position them at user-defined distances, yank and place pie slices, and create multiple linked pies. The presentation software package should allow log-log or semi-log scaling of business chart axes. Finally, it should be able to import .WK1 files, too.

⇨ Technical charts

Technical chart types should include box plots, contour plots, histograms, polar charts, spider plots, and surface plots. Options for scaling chart axes should include logarithmic scaling (base 10 or natural) and the use of multiple x- and y-axes. Curve-fitting options should include linear regression and polynomial or exponential curve fitting. The presentation software should be able to plot mathematical functions and save all data in a file.

⇨ Data handling

The data-handling facility should be able to import or export files that have one of the following formats:

> ➤ ASCII files (comma-delimited, tab-delimited, or fixed length)
> ➤ .DBF (dBase)
> ➤ .DIF (Lotus)
> ➤ SYLK
> ➤ .XLS 3.x
> ➤ .XLS 4.0 (Excel)
> ➤ .XQS (Quattro Pro)

It should be possible for you to import named data ranges, and you should be able to save such data ranges in a data sheet. You should be able to have, potentially, an unlimited number of data series in data sheets, as well as, potentially, an unlimited number of data points in each data series. Math functions should be included with data sheets. The data points in these data sheets should be transformable by functions.

Data linkages should include live links to external worksheets. It should be possible for presentation software to import charts from Harvard Graphics, Lotus 1-2-3, and Excel.

⇨ Chart editing & formatting

You should be able to edit text directly on charts. You should also be able to rotate charts and scale them to fit available space. Choose presentation software that lets you hide or display chart grids. Additionally, you should be able to create or import fill patterns and use them to put gradient fills in objects or slide backgrounds. Another chart editing and formatting feature that is quite nice to have is the ability to create chart legends that display calculated information, such as percentages.

⇨ Color handling

Color handling capabilities should include user-definable color palettes and pre-defined palettes. These palettes should contain as many as 16.8 million colors.

You should be able to use color for creating horizontal, vertical or angled gradient fills. You should also be able to apply a global color scheme to charts. Your presentation software should be able to handle Color PostScript.

⇨ Annotation

Chart annotations should include freeform labels and shadowed boxes. Text formatting should be fast, easy and flexible.

⇨ Illustration

Illustration tools should be able to draw arcs, curves and rounded boxes. They should also be able to draw lines, polylines, boxes and circles. The toolkit should include tools for putting objects in layers. Users should be able to align objects to baselines or to other objects, and you should be able to resize the objects or move them from front layers to back layers.

You should be able to zoom in on objects, break them apart or join them together. You should also be able to flip or mirror objects, and rotate them to any angle. It is also very convenient to be able to add arrows, comments, notes, labels, and pointers to illustrations.

You should be able to import/export files with the following formats:

➤ CGM (Computer Grahics Metafile)

➤ .DRW (Micrografx)

➤ .DXF (AutoCAD)

➤ EPS (.AI format)

➤ EPS

➤ .PIC (Lotus)

➤ .WMF (Windows metafile)

➤ WPG (WordPerfect Graphics)

You should be able to import/export these bitmapped file formats: .BMP, .CLP, .GIF, .IMG, .PCX, .TGA, and TIFF.

⇨ Presentation management

Presentations should be controllable by slide templates, including user-definable templates. It should be possible to re-use templates from existing displays. Slide presentations should be able to have multiple backgrounds for each presentation. It should also be possible to suppress the background of any slide.

The presentation manager should include a sorter for slides and slide titles. It should support cutting and pasting slides to the Clipboard.

You should be able to import text files with such formats as AmiPro, DCA/RFT, Microsoft Word (DOS and Windows formats), RTF, WordPerfect (DOS and Windows formats), and WordStar.

The presentation manager should help users create speaker's notes and handouts.

⇨ Electronic presentations

Electronic presentations should be able to include transition effects between images. They should be able to display multiple on-screen graphs, using a common slide background.

You should be able to control the duration and sequence of displays, and create standalone run-time screen shows.

Electronic presentations should support sound boards and MIDI and waveform files. Other features that they should have are support for animation, hyperlinks, and MIDI and waveform files. They should also support Autodesk .FLI and MacroMind Director files.

⇨ Hardcopy presentations

The hardcopy production facility should support film recorders such as Agfa (SCODL), Lasergraphics, Polaroid Palette, and PTI Montage. It should have communication software to link to custom slide production services such as Autographix, Genigraphics, and MagiCorp.

Color handling should include the abilities to convert colors to gray scales, to convert colors to pattern fills, and to invert the colors of text and backgrounds.

The hardcopy production facility should be able to share network printers. Printing options should include the ability to group multiple images on paper handouts, suppress backgrounds, and group multiple slides on a page.

⇨ Vendor support

Make sure that vendor support includes an on-line tutorial and on-line help. High-quality hardcopy documentation should be available. Vendors should offer free technical support and a BBS.

Desktop presentation software

The features that you should consider when you choose desktop presentation software are:

> Chart creation

> Data importing and exporting

> Audio

> Video

> Animation

> Clip art

> Text handling

> Illustration

> Output

> Presentation management

> Presentation features

> Vendor support

Data import and export, text handling, illustration, output presentation management, and chart creation are areas in which speed is especially important.

Creating charts

Make sure that your desktop presentation software lets you create many different charts, including bullet charts, 3-D charts, data driven-charts, and more. You should also be able to edit and format charts, using such operations as scaling and editing text directly on charts.

Data importing & exporting

Desktop presentation software should be able to import text and
graphics, including such standard text formats as:

- ➤ ASCII
- ➤ .RTF
- ➤ WordPerfect file formats
- ➤ Microsoft Word file formats
- ➤ .CHT
- ➤ .DBF
- ➤ Lotus 1-2-3
- ➤ .WK
- ➤ .XLS

Audio

Your desktop presentation software should support such audio devices
as Sound Blaster, PC Speaker, CD-audio, Ad Lib, and any Windows
MCI device. It should be able to import MIDI and .WAV audio file
formats. Sound-manipulation abilities should include synchronization
of sound with video, fadeouts and loops, and duplication and
recording of sound. You should also be able to trigger sound or play
several sounds at once. Desktop presentation software should also
support 16-bit stereo sound.

Video

Make sure your desktop presentation software supports such video
devices as video capture boards, videodisks (both CAV and CLV), and
any Windows MCI video device. You should be able to import any
MCI-compatible file format, as well as .AVI, .MDV or .DVI file
formats. Additionally, you should be able to edit video clips, doing
such operations as cropping and looping.

⇨ Animation

Integration of animation into desktop presentations should include capabilities for creating, editing, cropping and looping animations. Desktop presentation software packages should be able to import such animation files formats as .AVI/.FLC and .FLI/.MMM.

⇨ Clip art

Your desktop presentation software should include such clip art handling abilities as the ability to import standard graphics formats, such as .BMP/.DIB, .CGM, .PCD, .PCX, TIFF, and .WMF. It should supply large numbers of video clips, animation clips, sound clips and clip art images.

⇨ Text handling

Good text-handling ability is a must. It should be possible for you to add special effects to text, adjust kerning and leading, align text on a baseline, and rotate text.

⇨ Illustration

Presentation software should include illustration tools and manipulation tools that can align illustrations to a baseline or to an object, resize objects, and form groups of objects or break them apart.

⇨ Output

Presentation software should be able to make slides or overheads and send the resulting files to laser disks, videotapes, or printers.

Print options should include print previewing, conversion of colors to pattern fills or gray scales, suppression of backgrounds or gradients, and preparation of handouts or speaker's notes.

Presentation management

Presentation management, one of the key features of presentation software, should be able to offer multiple slide backgrounds during each presentation. It should also be able to suppress the backgrounds of individual slides. There should be pre-defined slide templates and multiple slide templates per slide presentation.

Presentation features

It should be possible for your on-screen presentations to include special effects, image overlays, multiple transitions per presentation, and hyperlinks to other slides or software applications. There should be a tool for annotating on-screen presentations.

Graphics software

This section tells you how to choose graphics software, screen capture and conversion utilities, 24-bit paint programs, 2-D drafting programs, image editing software, and illustration programs.

Screen capture & conversion utilities

You should consider these key areas when you choose screen capture and conversion utilities: screen capture and conversion features; image processing; file conversion; output; and vendor support.

✳ Screen capture and conversion features

Screen capture and conversion utilities should be able to capture full screens, active windows, client windows, user-defined rectangles, and areas that are drawn freehand. They should also be able to capture icons, icon captions, and windows indicated by the mouse pointer. Screen capture utilities should be able to capture full screens from ordinary DOS applications and protected-mode DOS applications. These utilities should also be able to capture screens after a specified delay.

Screen capture utilities should be able to write files to disk automatically, using various file formats including a default format. These utilities should be able to save captured screens and print them simultaneously. They should be able to capture any Windows screen resolution, and they should be able to capture at least 16.8 million colors.

✻ Image processing

The image processing faciltity should offer users numerous zoom levels. It should also be possible to reduce colored images to 256 gray-scale levels, to 16 gray-scale levels, or to black and white. Image-processing functions should allow cropping, dithering, edge tracing, flipping/mirroring, gamma correction, and adjustment of brightness/contrast. The facility should also support posterizing, image rotation, posterizing, sharpening, softening, and image inversion to a negative image. The image processing facility should include an image editor or paint facility.

✻ File conversion

Screen capture utilities should have file conversion facilities that can import/export numerous file formats, and batch process them. These formats should include .BMP, .CGM, .CLP, .CUT, .DRW, .DXF, EPS, all Fax formats, and GEM. File-conversion utilities should also be able to import/export .GIF, HPGL, IFF (Amiga), .IMG, .JPG (JPEG) and Lossy compressed formats. These utilities should also be able to import and export Macintosh file formats, all .PCX formats, PhotoCD (import), PM Metafile, RAS (Sun), all .TGA (Targa) formats, all TIFF formats, .WMF, and .WPG.

✻ Output

Screen capture and conversion utilities should be able to display full-screen images. Users should be able to specify image size and position. They should also be able to specify the number of copies to be output, as well as the resolution of output.

❋ Vendor support

Finally, publishers of screen capture and conversion utilities should offer on-line help, toll-free technical support, a BBS, and printed documentation.

⇨ 24-bit paint programs

Paint programs must have a broad range of tools for painting, image editing, text handling, output, and data import/export.

❋ Painting

Painting tools must be able to simulate airbrush, chalk, charcoal, crayons and felt-tip pens, oil and watercolor brushes, pens, pencils, and stamps. Users should be able to edit and save brush shapes, control the diffusion and rate of flow of brush marks, and use brushes to make calligraphic lines. They should be able to draw arcs, circles and ellipses, freehand curves, spline curves and polylines or polygons. They should also be able to blend and smudge colors and shadows, control the diffusion and thickness of lines, and fill colors by similarity.

Users should be able to work in separate color channels, using a variety of textures and patterns. They should be able to set transparency values and feather the edges of objects while cloning them. Finally, they should be able to make gradient fills, while being free to choose centers for radial fills and angles for linear fills. Users should be free to choose multiple colors for fills.

❋ Image editing

Image editing tools must include image processing features such as global anti-aliasing, embossing, tinting and washing, blurring, softening, sharpening, and the ability to change saturation. Image editing tools must also include a color picker or color editor that supports HSV, RGB, HLS, and CMYK color models. Users should be able to erase images, flip or mirror objects, and use a wide variety of selection tools. They should also be able to select lines of pixels or use a magic wand to select objects by color. They should be able to feather the edges of images, duplicate or crop sections, protect colors, and mask type.

Users should be able to paint beyond window boundaries, open multiple windows, and use the Clipboard for handling images.

✳ **Text handling tools**

Text handling should offer support for a wide range of fonts, the ability to size and style type, and the ability to cut, paste, and copy text. It should also support text rotation and anti-aliasing.

✳ **Output**

Painting programs should support pressure-sensitive digitizing tablets, film recorders, printers, scanners, and frame grabbers. Printing options should include user-specified resolution, size, margins, and dither patterns. It should be possible to fit images to pages and assign images to page positions.

✳ **Data import and export**

Users should be able to import or export file formats such as .BMP (DIB), EPS, .GIF, JPEG, .PCX, PICT (Macintosh format), .TGA, TIFF (Intel and Motorola), and .WMF.

⇨ **2-D drafting progams**

You should consider the following areas when you choose 2-D drafting software:

- ➢ Workspace management
- ➢ Data import/export
- ➢ Drafting tools
- ➢ Measurement
- ➢ Annotation
- ➢ Device support
- ➢ Vendor support
- ➢ Platform

✳ Workspace management

The purpose of workspace management facilities is to control drawing objects and drawing layers, panning and scrolling, selection of drawing entities, zooming, programming, and more.

Control of drawing objects should consist of hiding, locking, cutting, copying, pasting, and moving objects. Users should be able to select entities for further processing, using such selection criteria as logical conditions, entity type, or last entity chosen.

Control of drawing layers should include naming layers, hiding or locking layers, moving objects from one layer to another, and coloring layers. Control of layers should also include the ability to explode objects to other layers. The maximum number of drawing layers supported by 2-D drafting software ranges from the 20 layers supported by Micro Cadam Plus to the unlimited number of layers supported by AutoCAD.

Two-dimensional software packages offer several types of zooming: dynamic zooms that use a zoom window, zooming by a specified factor, choosing the previous zoom, and zoom all or zoom extents.

Users should be able to use screen menus and tablet menus. They should also be able to control their software, using interpreted or compiled scripts.

Other desirable workspace management abilities include redraws that are interruptible and that can occur in the background. Additionally, users should be able to have multiple windows open simultaneously.

✳ Data import/export

Two-dimensional drafting software must be able to import and export data files that are in .DXF (AutoCAD) format. They should also be able to import or export files in IGES format.

✳ Drafting tools

Drafting tools should include a 3-D modeler capable of draft-quality rendering. Drafting tools should include double lines and variable snap grids. Snap grids should be of three kinds: center/midpoint, tangent/circle quadrant, and perpendicular/nearest point.

Drafting tools should be able to fillet between lines, arcs, and curves. Users should be able to cross-hatch within complex boundaries (between lines and fillets, lines and arcs, and so on).

✳ Measurement

Two-dimensional drafting software should support associative dimensioning in which dimensions are treated as associative entities, not just as collections of lines. Measuring systems should support both rectangular and polar coordinates. The measuring system should use an isometric grid, with horizontal increments independent from vertical increments.

Two-dimensional drafting software should be able to measure angles, areas, and perimeters. It should support three systems of dimensioning: single, chained, and baseline.

Users should be able to assign attributes to symbols and generate bills of materials. Finally, 2-D drafting software should be able to read the following measurement data files: ASCII (fixed-length, comma-delimited, and tab-delimited), .WK1, and .DBF.

✳ Annotation

Annotation facilities should be able to import ASCII text files (fixed-length, comma-delimited and tab-delimited). These facilities should include a built-in text editor, too.

Users should be able to create or import hatch patterns and use solid fills.

✳ Device support

Printing options should include background printing, print preview, printing of selected drawing layers, and printing of specified attributes. Drawing sizes should be adjustable to fit the available page. It should be possible to print multiple copies.

❋ Vendor support

Two-dimensional drafting software should include on-line tutorials and on-line help. Vendors should offer toll-free support and have a BBS. Printed documentation should be available.

⇨ Image editing software

Image editing software is intended for editing and improving scanned-in photographs. The most important features of image editors are:

- ➤ Painting tools
- ➤ Data import/export facilities
- ➤ Image-processing facilities
- ➤ Image editing tools
- ➤ Image-management facilities
- ➤ Input device support
- ➤ Output device support
- ➤ Vendor support

❋ Painting tools

Painting tools should include an airbrush that lets users specify pressure, thickness and transparency. Image editing software should also include a brush that lets users specify thickness and transparency, define textures, edit brush shapes and save them, and use color-sensitive painting modes.

Users should be able to make linear and radial fills. They should be able to use more than two colors for fills. They should also be able to specify the transparency of fills.

Finally, users should be able to draw circles and ellipses, spline curves, and Bezier or freehand curves.

❋ Data import/export facilities

Image editing software should be able to interpret and render EPS files, and write them with or without a TIFF preview. It should be able to import or export such file formats as .IFF (Amiga), JPEG, Kodak Photo CD (import only), Macintosh formats, .PCX, Scitex CT, .TGA, and compressed TIFF.

✳ Image processing facilities

Image processing facilities should support at least four different color models: CMYK, HLS, HSV, and RGB. Users should be able to edit in RGB or CMYK mode. They should be able to reduce images from color to halftone, or from a larger number of colors to a smaller. Users should also be able to dither colors or balance colors, and correct colors and gray scales.

Users should be able to define palettes and edit colors, altering hue and saturation. They should also be able to balance grays, and select highlights, midtones and shadows. In addition, they should be able to resample images to a lower resolution, compress or resize them, skew them, or change perspective.

It should also be possible for users to posterize images or create negatives.

✳ Image editing tools

Image editing tools should help users select images and filter, clone, combine, or otherwise alter them. Users should be able to split images into separate CMYK color channels and view or combine these channels. They should be able to edit in CMYK color, using separate channels for masks.

Bitmap selection tools should let users select circles and ellipses, edit nodes, and expand selections based on color similarity. These tools should also let users select objects based on color, using a magic wand. Bitmap selection tools should help users to move, resize, or edit their selections.

Filtering of images should include adding noise, averaging, despeckling, embossing, blurring (Gaussian or motion), smoothing, edge enhancement, and user-defined filtering.

Image editing tools should help users combine objects by adding or subtracting, combining with a mask, or by anti-aliasing. Image editing tools should also allow flexible adjustment of tones for editing highlights, midtones, and shadows of images.

Finally, users should be able to create masks by using Bezier, freehand, or spline curves. They should be able to save masks as alpha channels.

✳ Image management facilities

Users should be able to search for image files by file name or type. Image management facilities should include a thumbnail browser for viewing images and evaluating possible changes. Users should be able to attach labels to these thumbnails.

Finally, image management facilities should include the ability to catalog, archive, delete, import, or export image files.

✳ Input device support

Image editing software should support pressure-sensitive digitizing pads, still video cameras, and scanners (through Twain). It should support calibration of all of these input devices, too.

✳ Output device support

Image editing software should support film recorders and printers. Print options should include printing trim marks, registration marks, stepscales, and negatives. Users should be able to specify emulsion orientation (up or down), halftone dot shape and frequency, print margins, and print resolution.

Image editing software should support calibration of all output devices.

Users should be able to do color separations, independently specifying the angle and frequency of each CMYK channel. It should be possible to print individual color plates and a black plate. The image editing software should be able to compensate for dot gain, generate black, and remove undercolors. It should be able to perform gray component replacement, too.

❋ **Vendor support**

Vendors should provide toll-free support, on-line tutorials and help facilities, a BBS, and printed documentation.

⇨ Illustration programs

The key criteria for choosing an illustration software package are the quality of its vendor support and the quality of its tools for:

➢ Illustration

➢ Object alignment

➢ Object manipulation

➢ Text handling

➢ Data export/import

➢ Output

➢ Color separation

➢ Vendor support

❋ **Illustration**

Professional illustration tools should use drawing primitives such as arcs, circles, ellipses, polylines, and polygons. Circles should be definable by center and diameter. Ellipses should be definable by center and two axes, or by axis and eccentricity.

Drawing tools should close curved paths automatically, be able to chamfer and fillet, and be able to do intelligent gradient fills. These tools should also support intelligent connecting lines.

Users should be able to measure distances in points and picas, feet and inches, and in the metric system.

❋ **Object alignment**

Alignment tools should be able to align objects to a baseline or to a page. They should also be able to snap objects to a grid or ruler, to a baseline or center, to an intersection or perpendicular, to an endpoint or midpoint, to a quadrant or tangent, or to the nearest point.

✳ Object manipulation

Object manipulation tools should be able to combine objects and break up combinations of objects. They should be able to clip a bitmap to an object, change perspective or warp an object, blend or extrude objects, and copy or reuse them.

✳ Text handling

Professional illustration software should support Adobe Type Manager. It should support also Adobe Type 1 and 2, Bitstream Speedo, and TrueType type fonts.

Type size should be adjustable to any value between 0.1 points and about three thousand points. Users should be able to align text on a baseline, and adjust kerning, leading, and tracking.

✳ Data export and import

Professional illustration software should be able to import or export files that have these formats: .BMP, .CDR (CorelDRAW file format), .CGM, .DRW (Micrografx Designer file format), EPS, .GED (Arts & Letters), and .GEM (GEM vector). It should also be able to import or export these formats: HPGL, .PCX, PhotoCD importing, PICT (Macintosh file format), .TGA, TIFF, .WMF (Windows Metafile), and .WPG (WordPerfect Graphics).

It should be possible for users to trace color bitmaps, export selected drawing objects, and select the size and resolution of exported objects.

✳ Output

Professional illustration software should be able to support screen shows.

Desirable printing options include the ability to break complex curves into segments, specify curve flatness (both for objects and globally), print trim marks and registration marks, and print margins, headers, and footers. Users should also be able to center images on the page and fit them to the available space, fit images to the available space, and print multiple images on one page.

Users should be able to select objects to print. They should also be able to specify the number of bands in the color and shadow gradients of images.

✳ Color separation

Color separation abilities should include black generation, ink correction, dot-gain compensation, undercolor removal, and specification of C,M,Y,K screen angles and frequencies. Users should be able to print step scales and separation labels.

Illustration programs should support TruMatch, Focoltone, and Pantone color-matching systems.

✳ Vendor support

Vendor support should include toll-free technical support, a company BBS or other on-line support, on-line help and tutorials, and printed documentation.

17

Choosing network software

THE network operating system that you choose, and the software that you choose for managing it, will have a big impact on your productivity. Here is how to choose this software.

Network operating systems

You should consider the following areas when you choose a network operating system:

➢ Architecture

➢ Scale of business operations

➢ Memory usage

➢ Network security

➢ Network printing

➢ Server management (local & remote)

➢ Network directory services

➢ Remote access

➢ Connectivity to hosts

➢ Network administration

➢ Auditing facilities

Architecture

Choose a network operating system that has a multi-user, multitasking, and multithreading architecture. You can get a network operating system that supports more than 1000 user connections per server, and more than 8 or 10 server connections per user, if you need it. You can also get a network operating system that supports a maximum file size of at least several gigabytes. The maximum number of file locks can be 100,000 or more, as can the maximum number of open files.

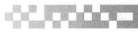

Choose a server that can support DOS files, Macintosh files, NFS files, OS/2 files, and Unix files.

➡️ Scale of business operations

Novell sells a network operating system for business operations that are in the range from small- to medium-size. It sells another network operating system for businesses that are in the range from medium- to large-size.

➡️ Memory usage

Your network operating system should offer dynamic memory allocation. Its maximum RAM size should be 4 gigabytes or more, as should the maximum cache size. Its system memory should be protected from access by applications.

➡️ Network security

Choose a network operating system that has C2 security certification. It should offer RSA public and private key encryption, detection and lockout of intruders, and access permission by user name and user group. Security features should also include access-control lists (ACLs) for each file. These should be stored with the files. Users should be able to limit the amount of hard disk space. Managers should be able to require password changes from time to time.

➡️ Network printing

Network printer-handling facilities should be able to assign priorities to jobs in printer queues. It should be possible to queue multiple printers on one queue, multiple printers to multiple queues, or multiple queues to a single printer. The network operating system should notify operators about any printing problems and it should notify them about job completion. It should automatically download the necessary printer drivers to any workstation that needs one. The

network operating system should also be able to manage remote
printer queues.

⇨ Server management

Local server-management software should display the number of bytes
and packets sent and received. It should also display an error and
system status log, cache statistics, hard-disk information, LAN-driver
information, and logical-disk statistics. Other displays should include
the number of open files, paging statistics, percentage of CPU use,
physical disk statistics, server data statistics, redirector statistics,
session statistics, and statistics of services from third-party servers.

Remote server-management functions should include facilities for
remote installation, remote upgrading, security for remote-console
sessions, and remote-console modem callback.

⇨ Remote access

The network operating system should provide a remote-access service
that has secure callback options. It should support asynchronous
telephone communications and dial-in using client/server
architecture. It should support ISDN, PAD, and X.25 protocols.

⇨ Network directory services

Network directory services should support globally distributed
databases and global name service.

⇨ Connectivity

Connectivity to hosts should include a remote 327x gateway option.
It should also support an asynchronous gateway option and an
asynchronous terminal emulation option.

⇨ Network administration

Network administrative functions should make it convenient to move objects in the directory service tree, copy inhibit (.COM or .EXE), hide directories and files, create, delete, or scan files, and grant permissions to users and groups of users.

⇨ Auditing facilities

Audit trails should show accesses to files and objects, show log-offs and log-ons, system shutdowns and restarts, system errors, and users and groups.

⇨ Network management software

Network management software must do tasks in these key areas:

- ➤ Inventory management
- ➤ Client PC monitoring
- ➤ Server monitoring
- ➤ Traffic monitoring
- ➤ Reporting and notification

All of these areas must be well integrated. Modules for each of these five areas should be able to share information with all the others, on the fly. All modules should have the same style of user interface.

⇨ Inventory management

The inventory management module should poll clients to see what hardware and software they contain. Polling ensures that the right versions of software packages are installed, hardware is compatible, and no equipment has been stolen. Inventory management software should be able to inventory both Macintosh and DOS/Windows hardware and software. It should also notify administrators of any hardware or software changes that have occurred.

Client PC monitoring

The client monitoring module should be able to determine the client address and the ID and type of the network interface cards for the client machine. It should also be able to learn the driver types used, as well as the version numbers of the drivers, the interrupts that they use, and the IPX and DOS versions that client PCs are running. The client monitoring module should also help administrators manage software on clients (and servers), keep track of licensing agreements, and make software upgrades throughout the network. It should monitor the functioning of client hardware, including screens, mice, keyboards, CMOS, ports, currently executing memory, recently executing memory, and other system hardware.

Server monitoring

Server monitoring software should keep track of server hard-disk size, available disk space, bad disk blocks, and disk and volume usage. It should notice and record changes in the server hardware configuration. It should also keep track of server CPU and memory usage.

Traffic monitoring

The traffic monitoring module should track overall network throughput. It should record the performance of the cache. It should also track and identify errors, including packet overflow and discarded packets.

Traffic monitoring software should record retries. It should also allow users to set thresholds for reporting.

⇨ Reporting & notification

The reporting and notification module should be able to assemble reports on the fly, and should be able to announce these to administrators by e-mail, fax, or beeper. It should also be able to display results graphically. Administrators should be able to set thresholds for reporting and notification. The reporting and notification module should be able to assemble a knowledge base about system performance over time. It should report password violations, log-ons at odd hours, and multiple stations that are logged on at the same time with the same name.

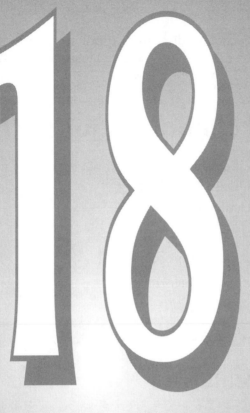

Choosing
miscellaneous
software

CHAPTER 18

THIS chapter discusses criteria for choosing communication software that has a graphic-user interface, fax software, and programmer's software.

⇨ GUI communication software

The most important criteria for choosing communication software with a graphic-user interface are its:

➤ Host features

➤ User interface

➤ File transfer protocols

➤ Network redirectors

➤ Program features

➤ Script language

⇨ Host features

Your comm software should include a facility for logging calls. It should also include dial-back capability. User access should be controlled by a password system.

⇨ User interface

The user interface for your comm software should support dragging and dropping of screen objects. It should have an icon bar that controls a dozen functions or so. You should be able to modify the icon bar, installing new functions or removing old ones.

It is very helpful if the user interface of your comm software displays modem lights. This way, if you have an internal modem installed, or an external one that has no lights, you will be able to diagnose comm problems, such as a loose cable, by watching comm lights.

⇨ File transfer protocols

Choose comm software that supports these protocols:

➤ CompuServe B\Quick B\B+,

➤ Kermit (with and without sliding windows)

➤ Xmodem-1K

➤ Xmodem-G

➤ Ymodem batch

➤ Ymodem-G batch

⇨ Network redirectors

Your comm software should support two network redirectors:
interrupt 14 and NASI.

⇨ Program features

You *can* get comm software that is carefully integrated with fax
software, so choose one that is. Choose a comm package that will let
you import or export ASCII telephone directories. The number of
telephone directories and the number of entries per directory should
be limited only by disk space.

Other features that you should seek are a built-in text editor,
password control of local operations, built-in context-sensitive help,
and a large number of pre-programmed modem setup strings.

⇨ Script language

Scripting languages are important for boosting productivity. They can
automate logging on to a host computer, automatically supplying user
IDs and passwords to the host. They can also automate such tasks as
downloading mail.

Your comm software will increase your productivity if it includes a scripting language facility that can watch what you do and automatically write scripts to do what you've just done. The scripting language should have about 300 verbs.

The package that you choose should include prepackaged "canned" scripts for logging on to services such as AT&T Mail, CompuServe, Genie and MCI Mail. WinComm Pro has a full set of these.

⇨ Fax software

Fax software should include tools for composing faxes. User interfaces for this software should offer context-sensitive help, toolbars, and mouse support. Fax software should be able to support many phone books that each have many entries. It should support Group 4 fax-transmission standards and support advanced Group 3 fax-transmission features, including 2-D encoding, binary file-transfer, and an error-correcting mode. Fax software should support all modem control standards. In particular, it should support CAS, Class 1, Class 2, FaxBIOS, and Send Fax modem control standards.

Fax software should include a variety of tools for composing and sending faxes. It should include a text editor, be able to access other text editors, and be able to compose cover pages and second pages. It should support bitmapped graphics so that faxes can include logos and signatures.

Users should be able to send faxes from within applications. They should be able to send selected parts of documents, and capture screens and send them as faxes. Users should be able to send faxes as a background activity, at times that they specify. It should be possible for users to broadcast faxes to multiple recipients, and to poll remote machines to see if faxing is possible or was successful.

Fax software should be able to intercept printer data and convert it to fax format. It should be possible for users to print data to fax software as they would to a printer.

➡️ Programmer's software

This section discusses two kinds of software: BASIC compilers and debugging tools.

➡️ BASIC compilers

Choose a BASIC compiler that has strengths in development environment, quality of executable programs, language features, and miscellaneous features.

✳ Development environment

Every BASIC language-development environment should include an executable program debugger. It should support step and trace execution, watch variables, and watch expressions, too. Users should be able to set breakpoints, break and resume execution somewhere else, and edit and resume execution after a breakpoint. Users should also be able to cut and paste between files and create executable files from within editors. The development environment should offer on-line help and mouse support.

✳ Executable programs

BASIC compilers should create standalone run-time programs. Programmers should be able to include on-line help in their programs.

✳ Language features

Language features should include such data types as bit arrays, byte variables, integers (signed and unsigned), long integers, double-long (8-byte) integers, and single-precision or double-precision variables. Data types should also include BCD variables, fixed-length strings, TYPE variables, and arrays within TYPE variables. BASIC compilers should also support huge arrays, constants, and initialized data.

✳ Miscellaneous features

Other desirable features are an in-line assembler, support for the AND, OR, and NOT bit operations, and libraries of functions for finance, graphics, charting, matrices, and statistics. Users should be able to require that all variables be declared. They should also be able to link subroutines written in assembler or other languages.

Conditional compilation should be possible, as should overlays, user-defined event handling and interrupt handling, and TSRs. Binary file access should be supported, as should ISAM file handling.

⇨ Debugging tools

Debugging tools come in four different flavors: analysis tools, application-level debuggers, system-level debuggers, and syntax checkers.

✳ Analysis tools

Analysis tools should validate pointers, identifying any that are corrupted or that do not have values assigned to them. Analysis tools should also detect local (stack) variables that are out of range, static (heap) variable that are out of range, and allocated (heap) variables that are out of range. Pointer checking should be done for applications and for libraries.

In Windows programming, analysis tools should be able to check local and global memory, trap fatal Windows errors, track object creation and deletion, support error-triggered callbacks, and check API parameters and return values.

Analysis tools should not change source code or require source code changes. They should not require additional libraries in order to work. Analysis tools should support C++, C, and assembler. Users should be able to direct the output from the analysis tool to printers, files, or to a second monitor.

✳ Application-level debuggers

Application-level debuggers should be able to set breakpoints and log breakpoints. They should also be able to set hardware breakpoints, including hardware I/O breakpoints. Application-level debuggers should be able to trace and execute code interactively. It should be possible for users to view and change variables or memory locations, browse data structures, and view registers. Application-level debuggers should also be able to display local and global heaps and perform automatic tracing in slow-motion. It should be possible to reverse execution, too.

✳ System-level debuggers

System-level debuggers should be able to do everything that an application-level debugger can do. In addition, they should be able to debug Windows VxDs, DOS device drivers, and DOS TSRs. System-level debuggers should also let users view and change calling parameters and returned parameters. They should let users debug or trace into interrupt vectors as well as trap calls to interrupts.

Other features that both system- and application-level debuggers should have are memory protection and support for class browsers and for debugging remote applications via serial ports or LANs. Both kinds of debuggers should support searching for functions, strings in source code, instructions, or other patterns in memory. After debugging runs, system-level debuggers should be able to do postmortem dumps.

✳ Syntax checkers

Syntax checkers should detect and warn about unreferenced values for symbols such as *typedef* and *macro*. They should also warn about unreferenced values for functions, global variables, automatic variables, and structure members. Syntax checkers should warn users about unused or repeated include files, too.

Detection of incorrect language usage is a key task for syntax checkers. They should alert users about empty *for* loops, *if/else* statements that do not match indentation, incorrect usage of bitwise operators, using assignment operators (=) where test operators (==) are needed, code that cannot be reached, lack of a condition in a *for* loop, and switch blocks that allow control to fall through to the next CASE statement.

Syntax checkers should identify functions that return undefined values, wrong data types, or the addresses of 'auto' data types. They should also check the parameters of calls to other functions. Finally, syntax checkers should also check the arguments of *printf* and *scanf* functions.

Appendix
Worker's
compensation
disability benefits

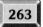

Table 1

Total Disability Benefit (1994)

States	Percent of Wages	Offsets
Alabama	66-2/3	
Alaska	80% of spendable earnings	Social Security, unemployment compensation, employer-funded pension, or profit-sharing plan
American Samoa	66-2/3	
Arizona	66-2/3	
Arkansas	66-2/3	Unemployment compensation, Social Security
California	66-2/3	Unemployment compensation. Social Security
Colorado	66-2/3	Social Security, unemployment compensation
Connecticut	75% of after-tax income	
Delaware	66-2/3	
District of Columbia	66-2/3	Social Security, employer-funded pension
Florida	66-2/3	Unemployment compensation, Social Security
Georgia	66-2/3	
Guam	66-2/3	
Hawaii	66-2/3	
Idaho	67	
Illinois	66-2/3	
Indiana	66-2/3	
Iowa	80% of spendable earnings	
Kansas	66-2/3	
Kentucky	66-2/3	
Louisiana	66-2/3	Social Security, unemployment compensation, employer-funded disability, federal workers' compensation
Maine	80% of after-tax average weekly wage	Employer-funded benefits, old age Social Security, unemployment benefits
Maryland	66-2/3	
Massachusetts	60	Unemployment compensation, pension, old age Social Security
Michigan	80% of spendable earnings	Disability, unemployment compensation, pension, old age Social Security retirement
Minnesota	66-2/3	Social Security after $25,000 paid for PTD
Mississippi	66-2/3	
Missouri	66-2/3	
Montana	66-2/3	Social Security
Nebraska	66-2/3	
Nevada	66-2/3	Social Security
New Hampshire	66-2/3	
New Jersey	70	Social Security
New Mexico	66-2/3	Unemployment benefits
New York	66-2/3	Social Security
North Carolina	66-2/3	
North Dakota	66-2/3	Social Security Disability and Social Security Retirement

Ohio	72-first 12 weeks 66-2/3 after 12 weeks; 66-2/3% if receiving Social Security Retirement benefits	Employer-funded benefits
Oklahoma	70	
Oregon	66-2/3	PT—Social Security
Pennsylvania	66-2/3	
Puerto Rico	66-2/3	
Rhode Island	75% of spendable income	
South Carolina	66-2/3	
South Dakota	66-2/3	
Tennessee	66-2/3	
Texas	70	
Utah	66-2/3	Social Security Disability and Retirement
Vermont	66-2/3	
Virgin Islands	TT—66-2/3 PT-75	PT—Social Security Disability and Retirement
Virginia	66-2/3	
Washington	60 to 75 depending on conjugal status	Social Security under age 65, Disability, Retirement
West Virginia	70	
Wisconsin	66-2/3	Social Security
Wyoming	TT—66-2/3 or SAMW	
F.E.C.A.	66-2/3 or 75	
Alberta	90% of weighted income	
British Columbia	75	
Manitoba	90% net (80% after 24 months)	Can. Pension Plan Disability Benefits & Disability
New Brunswick	80% of net average earnings for 39 weeks, 85% thereafter	Can. Pension Disability Benefits
Newfoundland	75% of net for first 39 weeks; 80% of net for claims longer than 39 weeks	Canadian Pension Disability Benefits
Northwest Territories	90% of net income	
Nova Scotia	75% of average gross income	
Ontario	90% of net average earnings	
Prince Edward Island	75	
Quebec	90% of weighted net income	
Saskatchewan	90% of net income	50% of Canada pension after 12 months
Yukon Territory	75	

Source: U.S. Chamber of Commerce. Analysis of Worker's Compensation Laws, 1994

Table 2

Benefits by Specific Injury

State	Arm at Shoulder	Hand	Thumb	First Finger	Leg at Hip	Foot	One Eye	Hearing One Ear	Hearing Both Ears
Alabama	$48,400	$37,400	$13,640	$9,460	$44,000	$30,580	$27,280	$11.660	$35,860
Alaska	No schedule. Benefits paid according to degree of whole person impairment.								
American Samoa	PPD benefits paid at 66-2/3% of wages for specified number of weeks, no maximum.								
Arizona	63,300	57,750	17,325	10,395	57,750	46,200	34,650	23,100	69,300
Arkansas	42,000	31,600	12,600	7,400	36,800	26,200	21,000	8,400	31,600
California	69,782	51,245	5,335	3,360	57,165	23,828	18,648	7,035	51,245
Colorado	31,200	15,600	7,500	3,900	31,200	15,600	20,850	5,250	20,850
Connecticut	110,032	88.872	33,327	19,044	81,995	66,125	83,053	18,515	55,016
Delaware	84,822.50	74,643.80	25,446.75	16,964.50	84,822.50	54,286.40	67,858	25,446.75	59,375.75
D.C.	211,901	165,717	50,937	31,241	195,600	139,229	108,667	35,316	135,834
Florida	No schedule. Benefits paid according to degree of impairment and loss of earnings.								
Georgia	56,250	40,000	15,000	10,000	58,250	33,750	37,500	18,750	37,500
Guam	70,000	53,000	12,750	7,000	62,000	43,250	35,000	13,000	50,000
Hawaii	150,072	117,364	36,075	22,126	138,528	98,605	76,960	25,012	96,200
Idaho	64,350	57,915	23,595	15,015	42,900	30,030	31,175	-	37,537.50
Illinois	213,876	135,456	49,905	28,517	196,055	110,504	114,068	38,473	76,946
Iowa	183,250	139,270	43,980	25,665	161,260	109,950	102,620	36,650	128,275
Maine	No schedule. Benefits paid according to degree of impairment.								
Maryland	153,200	127,539	17,000	6,800	153,200	127,539	127,539	11,775	127,539
Massachusetts	24,335.42	19,241.96	-	-	22,071.66	16,412.26	22,071.66	16,412.26	43,577.38
Minnesota	No schedule. Benefits paid according to degree of impairment and loss of earnings.								
Mississippi	48,750	36,562.50	14,625	8,531.25	42,656.25	30,468.75	24,375	9,750	36,562.50
Missouri	57,123	43,088	14,773	11,080	50,968	36,933	34,471	10,834	41,365
Montana	No schedule. Benefits paid according to degree of impairment, age, education, wage loss, and physical loss.								
Nebraska	59,625	46,375	15,900	9,275	56,975	39,750	33,125	13,250	—
Nevada	No schedule. Degree of disability determined in relation to whole man.								
New Hampshire	148,995	134,095	53,922	33,346	99,330	69,531	59,598	21,285	87,268
New Jersey	111,540	67,620	9,225	6,150	106,470	56,350	43,000	7,380	43,000
New Mexico	66,604	41,628	18,316	9,325	66,604	38,297	43,293	13,321	49,953
North Carolina	111,840	93,200	34,950	20,970	93,200	67,104	55,920	32,620	69,900
North Dakota	37,500	30,000	9,750	6,000	28,080	18,000	18,000	6,000	24,000
Ohio	108,450	84,350	28,920	16,870	96,400	72,300	60,250	12,050	60,250
Oregon	63,631	49,712	15,908	7,954	49,712	44,740	33,141	19,885	63,631
Puerto Rico	12,000	12,000	4,875	2,600	12,000	11,375	—	3,250	12,000
Rhode Island	28,080	21,960	6,750	4,140	28,080	18,450	14,400	5,400	18,000
South Carolina	90,257	67,693	26,667	16,410	80,001	57,436	57,408	32,821	67,693
South Dakota	67,600	50,700	16,900	11,830	54,080	42,250	50,700	16,900	50,700

State	Arm at Shoulder	Hand	Thumb	First Finger	Leg at Hip	Foot	One Eye	Hearing One Ear	Hearing Both Ears
Tennessee	71,194	53,395	21, 358	12,459	71,194	44,496	35,597	26,698	53,396
Utah	65,637	58,968	23, 517	14,742	43,875	30,888	42,120	17,550	35,100
Vermont	138,460	112,700	32,200	20,608	138,460	112,700	80,500	33,488	138,460
Virginia	90,200	67,650	27,060	15,785	78,925	56,375	45,100	22,550	45,100
Virgin Islands	62,040	50,760	22,560	22,560	50,760	33,840	54,990	33,840	50,460
Washington	71,280	64,152	25,660.80	16,038	71,280	40,896	28,512	9,504	57,024
West Virginia	67,253	56,044	22,418	11,209	67,253	39,231	36,989	25,220	61,648
Wisconsin	79,000	63,200	24,320	9,480	79,000	39,500	43,450	8,960	52,140
Wyoming	40,851	33,848	12,839	8,170	37,349	28,012	28,012	14,006	28,012
F.E.C.A.	401,691	314,143	96,560	59,224	370,791	263,931	205,995	66,948	257,494
Longshore Act	230,350	180,145	55,373	33,962	212,630	151,352	118,128	38,392	147,660
Indiana	48,000	34,000	6,400	4,000	41,000	27,000	27,000	8,500	34,000
Kansas	65,730	46,950	18,780	11,581	62,600	39,125	37,560	9,390	34,430
New York	124,800	97,600	30,000	18,400	115,200	82,000	64,000	24,000	60,000
Pennsylvania	202,130	165,155	49,300	24,650	202,130	123,250	135,575	29,580	128,180
Kentucky	No schedule. PP benefits paid at 66-2/3% of wages up to 425 weeks according to degree of disability.								
Louisiana	59,000	44,250	14,750	8,850	51,625	36,875	29,500	—	29,500
Michigan	127,775	102,125	30,875	18,050	102,125	76,950	76,950	Based on lost earnings	
Oklahoma	53,402.50	42,722	12,816.40	7,476.35	53,402.50	42,722	42,722	21,361	64,083
Texas	No schedule. Benefits paid according to degree of impairment.								

Source: U.S. Chamber of Commerce. Analysis of Worker's Compensation Laws, 1994

Bibliography

Ahlbom, A., M. Feychting, M. Koskenvuo, J. H. Olson, E. Pukkala, G. Schulgen, and P. Verkasalo. 1993. "Electromagnetic Fields and Childhood Cancer." *The Lancet*. 342 (8882): 1295-1296.

Allen, C. W., Jr. 1993. "Weight of Evidence Links Obesity, Fitness to Carpal Tunnel Syndrome." *Occupational Health and Safety*. November, 51-52.

Allen, Robert A. 1988. "User's perception of computer system response time." Ph.D. thesis. Clemson University.

Alsop, Stewart. 1993. "We all agree that groupware is good, but can it ever be delivered?" *Infoworld*. August 16. 15: 4.

Altman, Lawrence. June 5, 1988. "Study Links Risk of Miscarriage to Heavy VDT Use." *St. Paul Pioneer Press Dispatch*, from a *New York Times* article.

The American Heart Association Cookbook, Fifth Ed. 1991. New York: Random House Times Books.

"American National Standard for Human Factors Engineering at Visual Display Terminal Workstations." *ANSI/HFS 100*. 1988. Santa Monica, CA: Human Factors Society.

Analysis of Workers' Compensation Laws. 1994. Washington, DC: U.S. Chamber of Commerce.

Anderson, Alun. 1991. "Networks for thinking in cliques?" *Science.* August 2. 253, 505-507.

Anderson, Howard. 1991. "Network computing: A special report to management prepared by the Yankee Group." *Forbes.* May 27, 147: 147-151.

Andersson, G. B. J., R. W. Murphy, R. Oertengren, and A. L. Nachemson. 1979. "The Influence of Backrest Inclination and Lumbar Support on Lumbar Lordosis in Sitting." *Spine,* 4: 52-58.

Anthes, Gary H. 1993. "Geological survey speeds up map production." *Computerworld.* September 27, 27: 54.

Anzovin, S. 1993. *The Green PC.* New York: Windcrest/McGraw-Hill.

Assembly Engineering. November 1988, 30-33.

Austin, D. 1984. *Tone Up at the Terminal.* Verbatim Corp.

Baecker, Ronald. 1993. *Readings in groupware and computer-supported cooperative work.* San Mateo: Morgan Kaufman.

Barber, Raymond E. and Henry C. Lucas. 1983. "System response time, operator productivity, and job satisfaction." *Communications of the ACM.* 26: 972-986. November.

Barney, Doug. 1993. "Users trumpet notes for some applications: Groupware tool is better suited to documents, text than numbers." *Infoworld.* July 5, 15: 37-38.

Baron, R. 1979. *Varicose Veins: A Commonsense Approach to Their Management.* New York: Wm. Morrow and Co.

Barr, Christopher. 1992. "Are you talking to me? Workgroup apps to enhance collaboration." *PC Magazine.* December 8, 11: 29-31.

Baum, David. 1993. "Apple Open Collaboration Environment: combining personal communication with workgroup computing." *Infoworld*. May 31, 115: 53-54.

Beatty, William F. 1979. "Performance effects of system response time in human computer tasks." M.S. thesis. Virginia Polytechnic Institute and State University.

Bergman, Hans. 1981. *System response time and problem solving behavior*. Utrecht, The Netherlands: Psychological Laboratory, University of Utrecht.

Bermant, Charles. 1991. "Notes organizes Met Life's investment department." *PC Week*. October 14, 8: S27.

Bird, Jane. 1993. "Hard facts on software." *Management Today*. August. :57.

Boies, S.J., and Gould, J.D. 1971. "User performance in an interactive computer system." *Proceedings of the Fifth Annual Conference on Information Sciences and Systems*. Department of Electrical Engineering, Princeton University, New Jersey.

Bowen, Ted Smalley. 1993. "Aldus set to enter workflow publishing arena." *PC Week*. July 19, 10: 6.

Brady, J. 1986. "A theory of productivity in the creative process." *IEEE Computer Graphics and Applications*. May, :25-34.

Brennan, Laura.1992. "Groupware eases messaging, but beware of info overload." *PC Week*. October 26, 9: S29.

Bridges, Linda. 1992. "Groupware: what does it mean?" *PC Week*. October 26, 9: S3.

Brill, M. 1984. *Using Office Design to Increase Productivity: The BOSTI Study*. Buffalo, NY: Workplace Design and Productivity.

Brodeur, Paul. 1989. "Annals of Radiation. The Hazards of Electromagnetic Radiation. III. Video Display Terminals." *The New Yorker*. June 26: 39-68.

Brodeur, Paul. 1989. *Currents of Death: Power Lines, Computer Terminals, and the Attempt to Cover Up Their Threat to Your Health*. New York: Simon and Schuster.

Butler, T.W. 1984. "Computer repsonse time and user performance during data entry." *AT&T Bell Laboratories Journal*. July/August, 63: 1007-1018.

Byte. 1993. "Rolling the DICE." *Byte*. March, 18: 126.

Cafasso, Rosemary. 1992. "IBM mulls groupware strategy." *Computerworld*. November 23, 26: 1-2.

Carmel, Erran. 1992. "EMS speeds JAD sessions." *Computerworld*. May 11, 26: 1-2.

Carpal Tunnel Syndrome. Selected References. 1989. Cincinnati, OH: U.S. Department of Health and Human Services, Public Health Service, Centers for Disease Control, National Institute for Occupational Safety and Health.

Chaffin, D. B. 1973. "Localized Muscle Fatigue—Definition and Measurement." *Journal of Occupational Medicine*, 15: 346.

"Chained to His Desk." *Minneapolis Star Tribune*. July 12, 1994. p. 13

Chandler, Doug. 1990. "Buyers plunge in despite groupware debate." *PC Week*. May 14, 7: 121.

Clarkson, Mark A. 1993. "Hitting warp speed for LANs: High-speed networks promise the performance that collaborative computing needs—at a price." *Byte*. March, 18: 123-127.

Coffee, Peter. 1991. "PCs can promote cooperative problem solving." *PC Week*. September 9, 8: 58.

Coleman, Donald E. 1992. "Computer programs call meetings to order." *HR Focus*. August, 69: 10.

Collins, B. L. 1975. *Windows and People: A Literature Review—Psychological Reaction to Environments With and Without Windows*. Document No. C13.29/2:70. Washington, DC: NBS Building Science Series 70.

Comaford, Christine. 1993. "Integrated team processing comes of age." *PC Week*. January 18, 10: 52.

Computerworld. 1992. "Workgroup technology: typing technology to business objectives." *Computerworld*. March 23, 26: S3-11.

Cooley, D. and C. Moore. 1992. *Eat Smart for a Healthy Heart*. Hauppauge, NY: Barron.

Corbetta, Maurizio; Miezin, Francis M.; Dobmeyer, Susan; Shulman, Gordon L. et al. 1990. "Attentional modulation of neural processing of shape, color, and velocity in humans." *Science*. June, 248(4962): 1556-1559.

Costigan, M. 1991. "Employer Empowerment." *Business Insurance*, September 16: 57.

Crowley, Aileen. 1992. "Successful work groups need to overcome workers' tendencies toward individuality." *PC Week*. October 26, 9: S25.

Csikszentmihalyi, Mihaly. 1991. "Flow: the psychology of optimal experience." New York: Harper Perennial.

Damore, Kelley. 1992. "Multimedia firms aim for workgroups." *InfoWorld*. October 26, 14: 18.

Data Communications. 1992. "View from the top: industry leaders on networking's future; innovators offer opinions on everything from desktops to global nets." *Data Communications*. September, 21: 33-38.

Davisson, J. 1994. "Cutting Workers' Comp Costs." *Occupational Hazards*. February: 26-29.

Dayton, Doug. 1991. "Managers must seek a balance in data access." *PC Week*. October 14, 8: S37.

DeBakey, M. E., A. M. Gotto, L. W. Scott, and J. D. Foreyt. 1984. *The Living Heart Diet*. New York: Raven.

DeBusk, R. F., U. Stenestrand, M. Sheehan, W. L. Haskell. 1990. "Training Effects of Long versus Short Bouts of Exercise in Healthy Subjects." *American Journal of Cardiology*, 67 (4): 325-6.

DeMarco, T. and T. Lister. 1987. *Peopleware: Productive Projects and Teams*. New York: Dorset House Publishing.

Doherty, W.J., and R.P. Keliskey. 1979. "Managing VM/CMS systems for user effectiveness." *IBM Systems Journal*. 18(1): 143-163.

Duffy, Caroline A. 1992. "Pondering groupware's future; leaders: Nascent market is melting pot for future advanced technologies." *PC Week*. October 26, 9: S32-34.

Duncan, J. J., N. F. Gordon, C. B. Scott. 1991. "Women Working for Health and Fitness: How Much Is Enough?" *Journal of the American Medical Association*. December 18, 266 (23): 3295-3299.

Dunkle, John O. 1990. "Working well in a work-group environment." *Computerworld*. June 4, 4: SR31-33.

Dyson, Esther. 1990a. "Why groupware is gaining ground." *Datamation*. March 1, 36: 52-54, 56.

Dyson, Esther. 1990b. "Shearson's image of groupware." *Datamation*. April 1, 36: 61.

Dyson, Esther. 1991. "How to computerize a business conference." *Forbes*. April 29, 147: 143.

Dyson, Esther. 1993. "Tools won't help if you don't know what you're doing." *Computerworld*. March 22, 27: 33.

Easton, Annette; Easton, George; Flatley, Marie and Penrose, John. 1990. "Supporting group writing with computer software." *Bulletin of the Association for Business Communication*. June, 53: 34-38.

Edwards, Morris. 1992. "Some notes on groupware for LANs." *Communication News*. July, 29: 42.

Ellison, Carol. 1990. "Notes' graphics tools: can they get the job done?" *PC Computing*. March, 3: 107-109.

Eriksen, Warren J. 1966. "A pilot study of interactive versus non-interactive debugging." *TM-3296, System Development Corporation*. Santa Monica, California. December 13.

Foley, D. 1985. "The Chair-Sitter's Guide to a Better Bottom Half." *Prevention*. May: 92-109.

Folkers, K. 1986. "Contemporary Therapy with Vitamin B6, Vitamin B2, and Coenzyme Q10." The Priestley Medal Lecture Address. *Chemical and Engineering News*. April 21, 1986: 27-30, 55-56.

Fried, Robert. 1993. "What is theta?" *Biofeedback and Self Regulation*. March 18, 1: 53-58.

Galloway, L. 1919. "Office Management: Its Principles and Practice." *The Remington Office Manual*. New York: Ronald Press.

Gantt, James D. and Beise, Catherine M. 1993. "The public reacts to GDSS." *Byte*. March, 18: 118.

Garcia, Mary Ryan. 1991. "Lotus Notes untangles red tape at tax department: Switch from manual system lets agency answer taxpayers' questions in minutes." *PC Week*. October 14, 8: S28-30.

Geber, Beverly. 1990. "Groupware: altogether now." *Training: The Magazine of Human Resource Development*. September, 27: 79.

Geen, R. G. "Preferred Stimulation Levels in Introverts and Extroverts: Effects on Arousal and Performance." *Journal of Personality and Social Psychology*. 46: 1303-1312.

Gholamabbas, Ali. 1987. "The relationship between computer user attitudes and user perceptions of response time." Ph.D. thesis. United States International University.

Gibson, Steve. 1990. "Application response time is critical to productivity." *Infoworld*. May 21, 12(21): 28.

Gillin, Paul. 1990. "Group(ware) therapy: tips for success." *Computerworld*. November 5, 24: 109-112.

Goding, E. C. and J. J. Hacunda. 1993. *Computers and Visual Stress.* Charlestown, RI: Seacoast Information Services.

Goldhaber, M. K., M. R. Polen, and R. A. Hiatt. 1988. "The Risk of Miscarriage and Birth Defects Among Women Who Use Visual Display Terminals During Pregnancy." *American Journal of Industrial Medicine.* 13: 695-706.

Goulde, Michael. 1991. "Surveying groupware's competitive landscape: Lotus' Notes leads the field, but other products also meet users' needs." *PC Week.* October 14, 8: S5-9.

Grandjean, E., W. Hunting, and M. Pidermann. 1983. "VDT Workstation Design: Preferred Settings and Their Effects." *Human Factors.* 25(2): 161-175.

Grandjean, Etienne. 1987. *Ergonomics in Computerized Offices.* New York: Taylor & Francis.

Grant, E.E., and Sackman, H. 1966. "An exploratory investigation of programmer performance under online and offline conditions." *SP-2581, System Development Corporation.* Santa Monica, CA. September 2.

Grehan, Rick. 1992. "A shared resource access manager, part 1." *Byte.* August, 17: 279-284.

Greif, Irene. 1988. *Computer-supported cooperative work: a book of readings.* San Mateo, CA: Morgan-Kaufman.

Grieco, A. 1986. "Sitting Posture: An Old problem and a New One." *Ergonomics.* 29 (3): 345-3624.

Grossberg, M., Wiesen, R.A., and Yntema, D.B. 1976. "Experiments on problem solving with delayed computer responses." *IEEE Transactions on Systems, Man and Cybernetics SMC-6.* No. 3: 219-222. March.

Gullo, Karen. 1990. "Linked system aids joint efforts." *American Banker.* January 17, 155: 10.

Gullo, Karen. 1992. "New York banks stuff Lotus' suggestion box." *American Banker.* February 4, 157: 3.

Guynes, Jan Lucille. 1985. "Impacts of personality type and computer system response time on anxiety and user response time." Ph.D. thesis. North Texas State University.

Guyton, A. C. 1992. *Human Physiology and Mechanisms of Disease*. Fifth Edition. Philadelphia: W. B. Saunders.

Haavind, Robert. 1990. "Hypertext: The smart tool for information overload." Technology Review. November-December, 93: 42-50.

Haavind. Robert. 1990. "Groupware addressing need for productivity." *Electronic Business*. September 17, 16: 69-70, 72.

Hamilton, Rosemary. 1992. "Teamwork key to groupware success." *Computerworld*. August 19, 26: 1-2.

Hammer, W. 1989. *Occupational Safety Management and Engineering*. Englewood Cliffs, NJ: 50-51.

Hansson, T. 1986. "Prolonged Sitting and the Back." *Proceedings of the Conference: Work with Display Units*. Stockholm, Sweden: Swedish National Board of Occupational Safety and Health: 491-493

Harris, L, et al. Vol. I, 1978; vol. II, 1980. *The Steelcase Study of Office Environments*. Grand Rapids, MI: Steelcase Co.

Haubner, P., and S. Kokoschka. 1983. *Visual Display Units: Characteristics of Performance*. Amsterdam, 52 Bd. Malesherbes, Paris: International Commission on Illumination (CIE), 20th Session.

Herbert, L. A. 1992. "Body at Work." *Occupational Health and Safety*. October: 48-58.

Herbert, L. A. 1993. "Analytical Focus Reduces Anxiety Over CTD Claims." *Occupational Health and Safety*. April: 56-62.

HETA 90-013-2277. 1993. "Upper Extremity Musculoskeletal Disorders Among Newspaper Employees." *Los Angeles Times*. U.S. Dept. of Health and Human Services, National Institute for Occupational Safety and Health.

Higgins, Steve. 1992a. "Microsoft previews 19 work-group apps: building blocks seen targeting Notes." *PC Week*. October 5, 9: 1-3.

Higgins, Steve. 1992b. "Groupware '92 to spotlight PC electronic conferencing." *PC Week*. August 3, 9: 12.

Higgins, Steve. 1992c. "WordPerfect set to step up its groupware push." *PC Week*. August 31, 9: 1.

Higgins, Steve. 1992d. "Groupware: getting a grip on work-group computing; it's hard to pin down the definition." *PC Week*. October 26, 9: S1-3.

Hsu, Jeffrey and Lockwood, Tony. 1993. "Collaborative computing: computer-aided teamwork will change your office culture forever." *Byte*. March, 18: 112-118.

Huntington, L., T. Laeubli, and E. Grandjean. 1981. "Postural and Visual Loads at VDT workplaces, Part I: Constrained Postures." *Ergonomics*, 24: 917-931.

Husted, Bill. 1994. "Having hot-rod computer unnecessary for the work most users want to do." *Atlanta Journal and Atlanta Constitution*. March 20, Sec R, p 11, col 1.

IBM. 1982. "The economic value of rapid response time." White Plains, New York: IBM.

Ishii, Hiroshi. 1990. "Cross-cultural communication and computer-supported work." *Whole Earth Review*. Winter, :48-52.

Jackson, Susan A. 1992. "Elite athletes in flow: The psychology of optimal sport experience." Ph.D. thesis. University of North Carolina at Greensboro.

Jackson, Susan A. and Roberts, Glyn C. 1992. "Positive performance states of athletes: toward a conceptual understanding of peak performance." *Sport Psychologist*. June 6, 2: 156-171.

Johnson, Maryfran. 1992. "New groupware player (Xerox Corporation's Xsoft division)." *Computerworld*. November 23, 26: 45.

Jou, Jerwen and Harris, Richard J. 1992. "The effect of divided attention on speech production." *Bulletin of the Psychonomic Society*. July 30, 4: 301-304.

Karon, Paul. 1991. "Seybold consultants aim to form close electronic links with clients." *PC Week*. October 14, 8: S27-29.

Kellar, David. 1993. "NEC shows workgroup application system." *Infoworld*. April 26, 15: 47.

Kelsey, J. L. 1975. "An Epidemiological Study of the Relationship Between Occupations and Acute Herniated Lumbar Intervertebral Discs." *International Journal of Epidemiology*. 4: 197-205.

Khalil, T. M., E. M. Abdel-Maty, R. S. Rosomoff, and H.C. Rosomoff. 1993. *Ergonomics in Back Pain*, New York: Van Nostrand Reinhold.

Khan, Saad. 1993. "PIMs move to workgroup; efficiencies are multiplied by enterprisewide implementations." *PC Week*. October 11, 10: 105, 108.

Kilbom, A. 1987. "Short- and Long-Term Effects of Extreme Physiologic Inactivity—a Review." In *Work with Display Units*, B. Knave and P. G. Widebaeck, ed. North-Holland: Elsevier: 219-227.

Kim, James. 1994. "Intel to bring users face to face." *USA Today*. January 24, 2B, col. 4.

King, J. A. 1993. "Economy Class Syndrome." *Endless Vacations*. Sept/October: 16, 103.

Kirkpatrick, David. 1992. "Here comes the payoff from PCs." *Fortune*. March 23, 125: 93-100.

Kirkpatrick, David. 1993a. "Mac vs. Windows." *Fortune*. October 4. :107-114.

Kirkpatrick, David. 1993b. "Groupware goes boom." *Fortune*. December 27, :99-106.

Kolowich, Michael. 1991. "Lessons from the baseball dugout for work-group computing." *PC Computing*. August, 4: 66.

Kotkin, Joel. 1994. "Commuting via information superhighways." *The Wall Street Journal*. January 27.

Kramer, Matt. 1992. "E-mail may hold key to groupware's future." *PC Week*. October 26 : S20.

Krieger, Roy. 1994. "On the Line." *ABA Journal*. January: 40-45.

Kroemer, K., H. Kroemer, K. Kroemer-Elbert. 1994. *Ergonomics*. Englewood Cliffs, NJ: Prentice-Hall: 444.

Kurzwell, Raymond. 1993. *The 10 Percent Solution*. New York: Crown Publishers.

Laberge, David. 1990. "Thalmic and cortical mechanisms of attention suggested by recent positron emission tomographic experiments." *Journal of Cognitive Neuroscience*. Fall, 2(4): 358-372.

Lambert, G. N. 1984. "A comparative study of system response time on program developer productivity." *IBM Systems Journal*. 23(1): 36-43.

LaPlante, Alice. 1992. "Group(ware) therapy." *Computerworld*. July 27, 26: 71-74.

LaPlante, Alice. 1993. "Taligent electronic bulletin board is a workhorse: groupware aids project coordination, act as a database, reinforces corporate culture." *Infoworld*. May 10, 15: 72.

Larson, Arthur. 1988. "Tensions of the Next Decade." In *New Perspectives in Workers' Compensation*, J. F. Burton, ed. Ithaca, NY: ILR Press, Cornell University.

Leffingwell, W. H. 1917. *Scientific Management*. New York: A. H. Shaw Co.

Leutner, Detlev and Gerd Schumacher. 1990. "The effects of different on-line adaptive response time limits on speed and amount of learning in computer-assisted instruction and intelligent tutoring." *Computers in Human Behavior*. 6(1)

Lewis, Jamie. 1993. "Workgroup apps fill the demand for flexibility." *PC Week*. March 15, 10: 44.

Lindbohm, M. L., M. Hietanen, P. Kyyroenen, M. Sallmen, P. V. Nandelstadh, H. Taskinen, M. Pekkarinen, M. Ylikoski, and K. Hemminke. 1992. "Magnetic Fields of Video Display Terminals and Spontaneous Abortions." *American Journal of Epidemiology*. 136 (9): 1041-1051.

Lindbohm, M. L., P. Kyyroenen, M. Hietanen, and M. Sallmen. 1993. "The Authors Reply." *American Journal of Epidemiology*. 138 (10): 903-905.

Lockwood, Russ. 1990. "The electronic office: who will have one, how will it work, where will you fit in." *Personal Computing*. May 25, 14: 74, 76, 78, 81-82.

Mandel, A. C. 1981. "The Seated Man (Homo Sedans)." "The Seated Work Position." "Theory and Practice." *Applied Ergonomics*. 12(1): 19-26.

Mantelman, Lee. 1992. "Workflow: improving the flow of corporate data." *Infoworld*. June 29, 14: 46-48.

Mantelman, Lee. 1993. "Workflow application tools: smart strategies for automating the way people and businesses work." *Infoworld*. February 22, 15: 56, 61.

Manzi, Jim P. 1992. "The productivity MacGuffin." *Byte*. August, 17:360.

Marsh & McLennan Protection Consultants, 1983. *Occupationally Related Hand/Wrist and Arm Syndromes*.

McCarthy, Vance. 1991. "Apple's System 7 casts lure for work-group computing environments." *PC Week*. May 20, 8: 14.

McGowan, Robert W.; Pierce, Edgar, F.; Jordan, David. 1992. "Differences in precompetitive mood states between black belt ranks." *Perceptual and Motor Skills*. August, 75(1): 123-128.

Meier, Barry. 1991. "UL Safety Standards Questioned." *Minneapolis Star Tribune*, April 18. From the *New York Times*.

Merchant, Asit V. 1991. "Workstation allocation schemes for response time improvement in a multiserver PC LAN." M.S. thesis. New Jersey Institute of Technology, Department of Electrical and Computer Engineering.

Meyer, E.; Ferguson, S. S.; Zatorre, R. J.; Alivisatos, B. et al. 1991. "Attention modulates somatosensory cerebral blood flow response to vibrotactile stimulation as measured by positron emission tomography." *Annals of Neurology*. April 29, 29(4): 440-443.

Miastkowski, Stan. 1993. "E-Quip: LAN paper management." *PC Magazine*. May 11 :12:50.

Miller, G. A. 1956. "The magical number seven, plus or minus two: some limits on our capability of processing information." *Psychological Review*. 63: 81-97.

Miller, Michael. 1986. "In this futuristic office, intimacy exists between workers separated by 500 miles." *The Wall Street Journal*. June 27 :31: 29.

Miller, Michael J. 1993. "No computer is an island." *PC Magazine*. July, 12: 81-83.

Minneapolis Star Tribune, September 20, 1988 (from The Washington Post).

Morgan, S. 1991. "Most Factors Contributing to CTS Can Be Minimized, If Not Eliminated." *Occupational Health and Safety*, October: 47-54.

Morrissey, Jane. 1991. "Work-flow computing will grow over 4-year period, study says." *PC Week*. December 9, 8: 129.

Mulloy-Steinborn, Jean M. 1993. "Affective and cognitive effects on response time to a computer administered version of the Eysenck personality questionnaire." Ph.D. thesis. Fordham University.

Musich, Paula. 1990. "WordPerfect Office taps into EasyLink." *PC Week*. June 11, 7: 5.

National Academy Press. 1983. "Display Work and Vision." *Report of the Panel on Impact of Video Viewing and Vision of Workers*. Washington, DC: NAP.

Nethery, Kee. 1993. "AOCE: Apple's plan for groupware." *Macworld*. November, 10: 165-168.

Newell, A. F. and Alistair Y. Cairns. 1993. "Designing for Extraordinary Users." *Ergonomics in Design*. Santa Monica, CA: Human Factors Society. October: 10-16.

Noidin, M. and V. H. Frankel. 1989. *Basic Biomechanics of the Musculoskeletal System. Second Edition*. Malvern, PA: Lem & Febiger.

Nye, Peter. 1994. "Grassroots Movement Seeks to Ground Electromagnetic Fields." *Public Citizen*. 14 (1): 18-31.

Oak Ridge Associated Universities. 1992. "Health Effects of Low Frequency Electric and Magnetic Fields." For *The Committee on Interagency Radiation Research and Policy Coordination (CIRRPC), Contract DE-AC05-760R00033 with the U.S. Department of Energy*. Pub. No. 029-000-00443-9. Washington, DC: U.S. Government Printing Office.

Occupationally Related Hand/Wrist and Arm Syndromes. 1983. Marsh & McLennan Protection Consultants.

Orleans, C. T. and J. Slade, ed. 1993. *Nicotine Addiction: Principles and Management*. New York: Oxford University Press.

Ornish, D. 1992. *Dr. Dean Ornish's Program for Reversing Heart Disease*. New York: HarperCollins.

Pascarelli, E. and D. Quilter. 1994. *Repetitive Strain Injury*. New York: John Wiley & Sons.

Pascarelli, E. F. and J. J. Kella. 1993. "Soft-Tissue Injuries Related to Use of the Computer Keyboard." *Journal of Occupational Medicine*. Vol. 35 (5), May: 552-532.

PC World. 1993. "LotusWorld to highlight progress in work-group computing." *PC World*. April, 11: L4.

Pearce, B. 1992. "Products to Relieve or Prevent VDU Health Problems: Exploitation, Placebos, or Prophylaxis?" In *Work with Display Units 92*. H. Luczak, A. Cakir, and G. Cakir, ed. North Holland: Elsevier Science Publishers: 500-506.

Perkins, S., M.D. 1992. *Gastrointestinal Health*. New York: HarperCollins.

Pinsky, M. A. 1993. *The Carpal Tunnel Syndrome*. New York: Warner Books.

Potter, J. D., M.L. Slattery, R. M. Bostick, and S.M. Gapstor. 1993. "Colon cancer, a review of the epidemiology." *Epidemiology Reviewed*, 15(2):499-545

Preston, Alyson. 1992. "As use of groupware increases, remote access, speed and security emerge as critical issues." *PC Week*. October 26, 9: S21.

Privette, Gayle and Bundrick, Charles M. 1991. "Peak experience, peak performance, and flow: correspondence of personal descriptions and theoretical constructs. A special issue: Handbook of Self-Actualization." *Journal of Social Behavior and Personality*. 6(5): 169-188.

Rabkin, Barry. 1993. "'Groupware' helps insurers handle catastrophic claims." *National Underwriter Property and Casualty-Risk and Benefits Management*. September 27, :74, 78.

Radosevich, Linda. 1993. "Vendors unite to promote workflow." *Computerworld*. August 2, 27: 16.

Rash Jr., Wayne. 1990. "The growth of groupware." *Byte*. November, 15: 89-92.

Raskin, Robin. 1993. "For the good of the group?" *PC Magazine*. January 12, 12: 30.

Rivera, Julio C. 1992. "An empirical study of the effect of system response time and task complexity on user decision quality." D.B.A. thesis. Mississippi State University, College of Business and Industry.

Robinson, Susan Carol. 1991. "MCI boosts its own communication with adoption of Notes." *PC Week*. October 14, 8: S28-30.

Rooney, Paula. 1993. "Ad agency gets creative with workflow technology." *PC Week*. September 20, 10: 83, 95.

Rosenblum, M., ed. 1973. *Compendium on Workmen's Compensation*. Washington, DC: National Commission on State Workmen's Compensation Laws.

Ryan, P., M. W. Lee, J. B. North, A. J. McMichael. 1992. "Risk Factors for Tumors of the Brain and Meninges: Results from the Adelaide Adult Brain Tumor Study." *International Journal of Cancer*. 51 (1): 20-27.

Sackman, H., Eriksen, W. J., and Grant, E. E. 1968. "Exploratory experimental studies comparing online and offline programming performance." *Communications of the ACM*. January, 11(1): 3-11.

Saffo, Paul. 1993. "The future of 'virtual' computer conferencing looks as clear as MUD." *PC Computing*. January, :104.

Sanders, Jenny. 1992. "Groupware shipments to double through 1993." *PC Week*. November 30, 9: 163.

Sandler, Harold and Joan Vernikos. 1986. *Inactivity: Physiological Effects*. New York: Academic Press.

Sauter, S. L., Schliefer, L. M., and S. J. Knutson. 1991. "Work Posture, Workstation Design, and Musculoskeletal Discomfort in a VDT Data Entry Task." *Human Factors*. 32: 151-167.

Sauter, S., M. Dainoff, and M. Smith. 1990. *Promoting Health and Productivity in the Computerized Office: Models of Successful Ergonomic Interventions*. New York: Taylor & Francis.

Schrage, Michael. 1990. *Shared Minds*. New York: Random House.

Schrage, Michael. 1991. "Computer tools for thinking in tandem." *Science*. August 2, 253: 505-507.

Schrage, Michael. 1993. Trying groupware on for (down) size. *Computerworld*. August 30, 27: 33.

Schuler, Michael. 1992. "Baby thought update." *Computers in Libraries*. December, 12(11): 56.

Schwabach, Bob. 1993. "Word processors offer many new features." *Star Tribune*. November 18, 2D, col. 1.

Seymour, Jim. 1991. "Tools help virtual work groups keep in touch." *PC Week*. April 29, 8: 65.

Sherer, Paul M. 1990. "Microsoft to debut office-linking spec." *PC Week*. December 10, 7: 1-3.

Sherer, Paul M. 1992. "Consortium plans to promulgate spec for multiuser DOS." *PC Week*. November 9, 9: 84.

Sherman, Stratford. 1993. "How to bolster the bottom line." *Fortune.* Autumn, 127(7): 15-28.

Shotton M. A. 1989. *Computer Addiction?* New York: Taylor & Francis.

Shukovsky, Sam. 1991a. "Team players gain optimal benefits from groupware." *PC Week.* October 14, 8: S11-13.

Shukovsky, Sam. 1991b. "GM links European operations with Notes." *PC Week.* October 14. : S29.

Simon, Barry.1991. "Tracking the minutes that groups spend on a project." *PC Magazine.* August, 10: 50.

Smith, A. 1989. "A Review of the Effects of Noise on Human Performance." *Scandinavian Journal of Psychology.* 30: 185-206.

Smith, Jerd. 1992. "New groupware lets company create collective consciousness." *Denver Business Journal.* June 5, 43: 19-21.

Snyder, H. 1986. "Screen Visibility Requirements and Criteria." In *The Ergonomic Payoff.* R. Lueder, ed. New York: Holt, Rinehart and Winston. 64-79.

Sommerich, L. M., J. D. McGlothlin, and W. S. Marras. 1993. "Occupational Risk Factors Associated with Soft Tissue Disorders of the Shoulder: A Review of Recent Investigations in the Literature." *Ergonomics.* 36 (6): 697-717.

Stein, Irene. 1983. "Relation between user think time and response time in an interactive system." M.S. thesis—Virginia Polytechnic Institute and State University.

Steinberg, Don. 1990. "How does Notes handle security?" *PC-Computing.* March, 3: 117-119.

Steinmann, M. 1989. *The American Medical Association Guide to Back Care.* New York: Random House.

Stinson, Craig. 1993. "Boost productivity by limiting Windows options; fail-safe tips to cut back on workgroup confusion." *PC-Computing.* September, 6: 298-302.

Sussman, S. and Dr. Ernest Loewenstein. 1993. *Total Health at the Computer*. Barrytown, New York: Station Hill Press.

Swanson, N. G., and S. L. Sauter. 1993. "The Effects of Exercise on the Health and Performance of Data Entry Operators." *In Work With Display Units 92*. A. Cakir and G. Cakir, ed. North Holland: Elsevier Science Publishers: 288-291.

Taber, Mark. 1992. "Can OfficeVision take off with Notes? Host-based integrated office systems and desktop personal productivity are linking with new high-flying work group products." *Datamation*. February 15, 38: 65-68.

Technology & Learning. 1992. "Groupware goes to school: New tools to promote group activity and learning." *Technology & Learning*. February, 12: 80-84.

Thadhani, A. J. 1981. "Interactive user productivity." *IEEE Computer Graphics and Applications*. 20(4): 407-423.

The Economist. 1990. "A curriculum for change." *The Economist*. June 16, 315: S11-S14.

The Society for Environmental Graphic Design. The Americans with Disabilities Act (ADA) White Paper. SEGA, 47 Third St., Cambridge, MA 02141.

Tichauer, E. R. 1973. *The Industrial Environment—Its Evolution and Control*. Washington, DC: National Institute for Occupational Safety and Health, Department of Health, Education, and Welfare. 138-139.

Tichauer, G. R. 1978. *The Biomechanical Basis of Ergonomics*. New York: Wiley & Sons.

Ulrich, R. 1984. "View Through a Window May Influence Recovery from Surgery." *Science*. 224 (4647). 420-421.

United States. National Bureau of Standards. 1978. "Guidelines for the measurement of interactive computer service response time and turn around time." Washington, DC.: Department of Commerce, National Bureau of Standards.

University of Utrecht. 1982. "The influence of system response time and memory load on problem solving behavior." Utrecht, The Netherlands: Psychological Laboratory, University of Utrecht.

U.S. Chamber of Commerce. 1993. "Analysis of workers' compensation laws." Washington, D.C.

VDT News. 1992. January/February, : 3, 10.

Vizard, Michael. 1993a. "Microsoft talks groupware options: looks to eradicate groupware applications." *Computerworld.* May 24, 27: 4.

Vizard, Michael. 1993b. "Power to the people (integration problems using groupware)." *Computerworld.* August 16, 27: 85-87.

Vizard, Michael. 1993c. "Vendors back Borland plan: Apple, MCI, WordPerfect to support groupware framework." *Computerworld.* September 20, 27: 8.

Von Simson, Charles. 1990. "It's time to grow up." *Computerworld.* March 12, 24: 37-39.

Weinstein, J. 1967. *Industrial Revolution and the Common Law: Big Business and the Origins of Workmen's Compensation.* 8 Lab.Hist.: 146.

White, A. 1990. *Your Aching Back.* New York: Simon & Schuster.

Whitehead, Roger. 1991. "Right hemisphere processing superiority during sustained visual attention. A special issue: The University of Oregon Center for Cognitive Neuroscience of Attention." *Journal of Cognitive Neuroscience.* Fall, 3(4): 329-334.

Wilke, John R. 1993. "Computer links erode hierarchical nature of workplace culture." *The Wall Street Journal.* December 9, A1, col 1, A7, col 1.

Willey, David. 1993. "Star tech (factors to consider when investing in information technlogy)." *Journal of Business Strategy.* July-August, 14: 52-54.

Winkel, J. 1987. "On the Significance of Physical Activity in Sedentary Work. In *Work with Display Units 86*. B. Knave and G. Widebaeck, ed. North Holland: Elsevier Science Publishers: 229-235.

Wohl, Amy D. 1992. "Groupware: collaborative computing comes of age." *Office Technology*. January, 26: 10-12.

Woodworth, R.S. 1938. "Experimental Psychology." New York: Henry Holt and Company.

Zacharkow, D. 1990. "The Problems with Lumbar Support." *Physical Therapy Forum*. IX, 35, September. 10: 2-5.

Zacharkow, D. 1994. "The Overlooked Factor in Carpal Tunnel Syndrome." *Advance*. May 16.

Index

Boldface page numbers refer to art

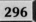

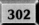

About the authors

Baird Peterson works as a software development contractor for businesses ranging from startup ventures to Fortune 500 companies. He is a contributing writer for *ComputerUser* and reviews educational computer software for magazines such as *Minnesota Parent*. Dr. Peterson received his Ph.D. from the University of Minnesota and has previously written books on the subjects of UNIX System V and XENIX.

Richard Patten is an expert on the complex interactions between people and machines. He designs CAD facilities for 3M, a Fortune 500 company, and has performed other duties for that company ranging from critiquing new product designs to analyzing accidents. Dr. Patten is also an editorial consultant for *Human Factors*, a journal about machine/people interaction, and is 1 of only 25 board-certified human factors experts in the United States. He received his Ph.D. from the University of Iowa and has previously published in scientific journals.